THE
CARNIVORE
CODE COOKBOOK

DISCOVER THE SECRETS OF SUSTAINABLE, NOURISHING MEAT-FOCUSED MEALS: FROM BEGINNER CARNIVORE TO MEAT MASTER.

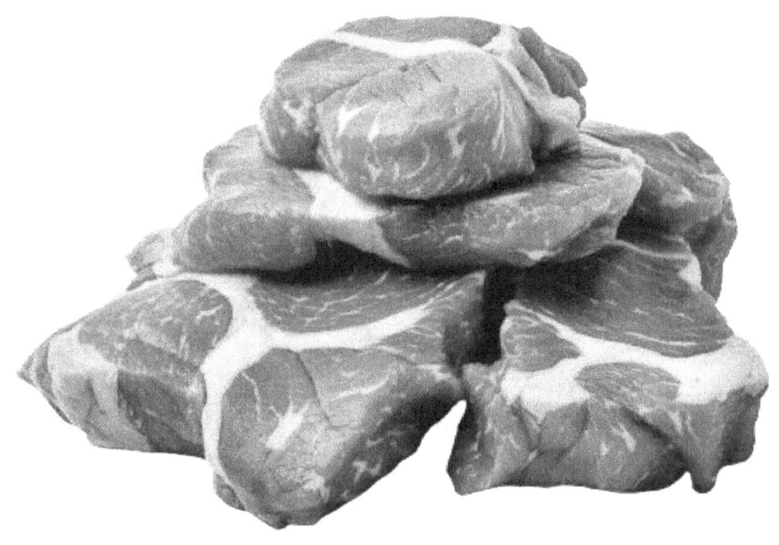

Nicole Crawford

COPYRIGHT

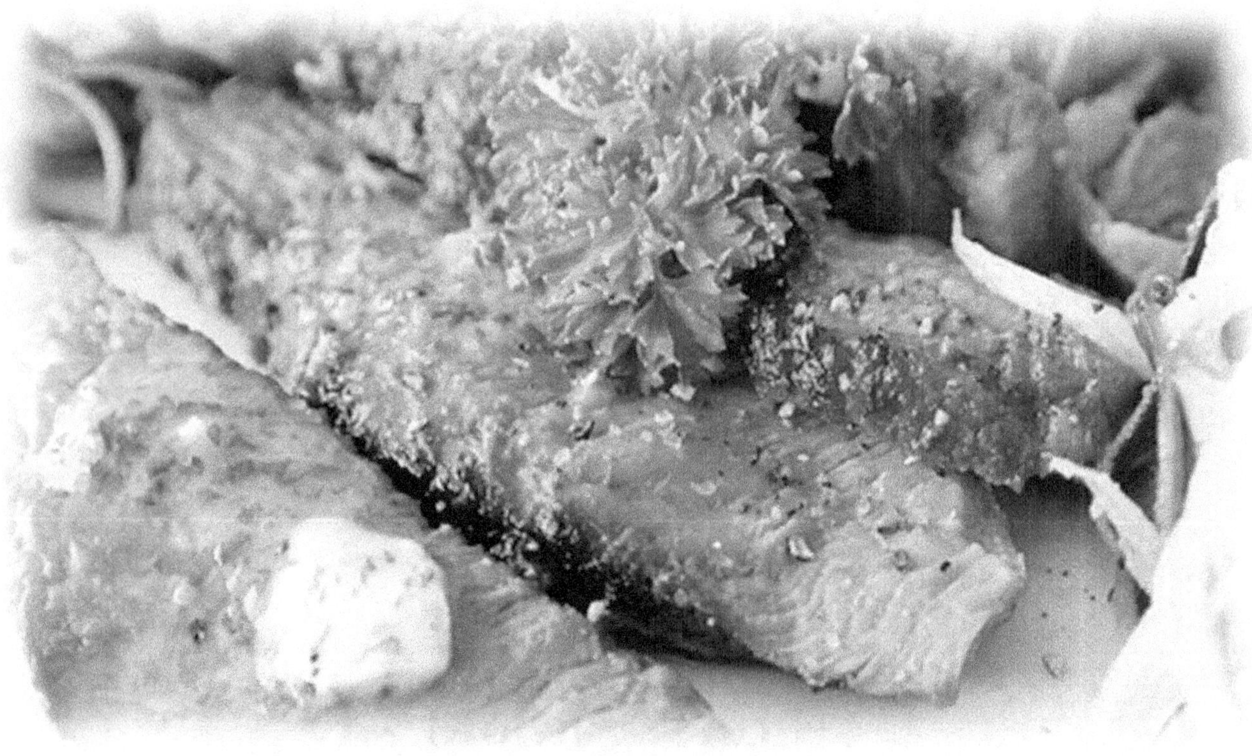

TABLE OF CONTENTS

CHAPTER 1: Introduction to the Carnivore Diet

- **What is the Carnivore Diet?**
- **The History and Evolution of Carnivore Eating**
- **Benefits and Potential Drawbacks**

CHAPTER 2: Understanding the Carnivore Diet

- **The Science Behind Carnivore Eating**
- **Nutritional Considerations and Health Impacts**
- **Common Myths and Misconceptions**

CHAPTER 3: The Essentials of the Carnivore Diet

- **Key Foods and Ingredients**
- **Understanding Meat Quality and Sources**
- **Organ Meats and Their Importance**

CHAPTER 4: The Carnivore Diet Rules

- **Do's and Don'ts of the Carnivore Diet**
- **Understanding Macros and Micros**
- **Hydration and Electrolyte Balance**

CHAPTER 5: Getting Started with the Carnivore Diet

- **Setting Up Your Carnivore Kitchen**
- **Shopping List and Pantry Essentials**
- **Transitioning to a Carnivore Diet**

CHAPTER 6: Carnivore Diet Styles and Recommendations

- **Different Approaches to Carnivore Eating**
- **Tailoring the Diet to Your Needs**
- **Recommendations for Optimal Health**

- **Mastering the Art of Meat Preparation**
- **Grilling, Smoking, and Sous Vide**
- **Making the Most of Leftovers**

- **Daily and Weekly Meal Plans**
- **Tips for Eating Out and Social Situations**
- **Portion size and frequency**
- **Tips for grocery shopping and meal prep**
- **How to Handle Cravings and Cheat Days**

- **Performance and Recovery on a Carnivore Diet**
- **Specific Considerations for Athletes**

CONCLUSION AND MOVING FORWARD

BONUS

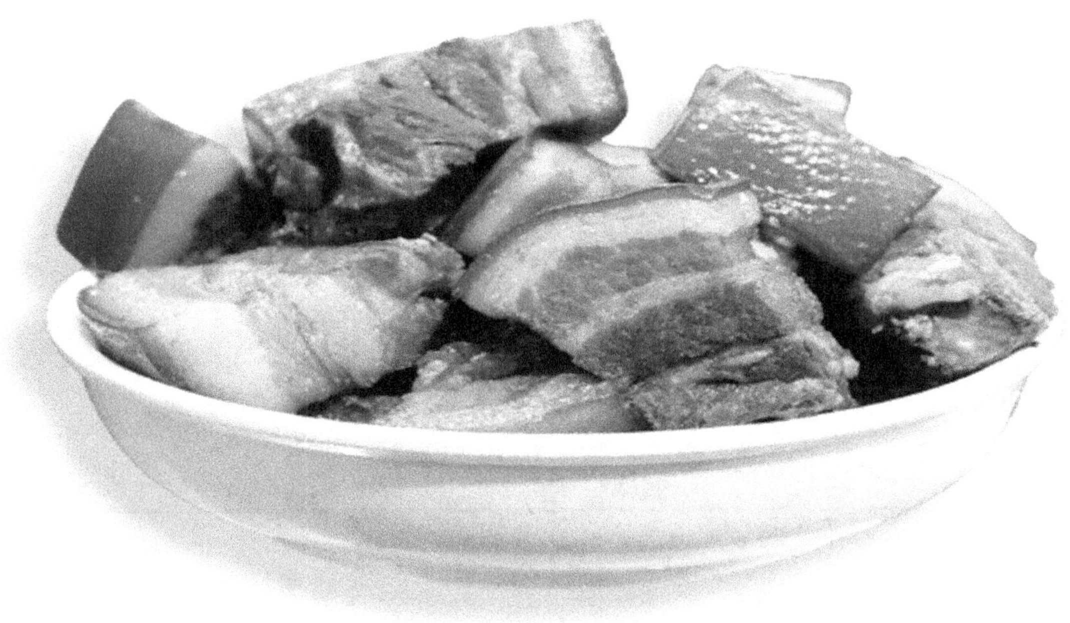

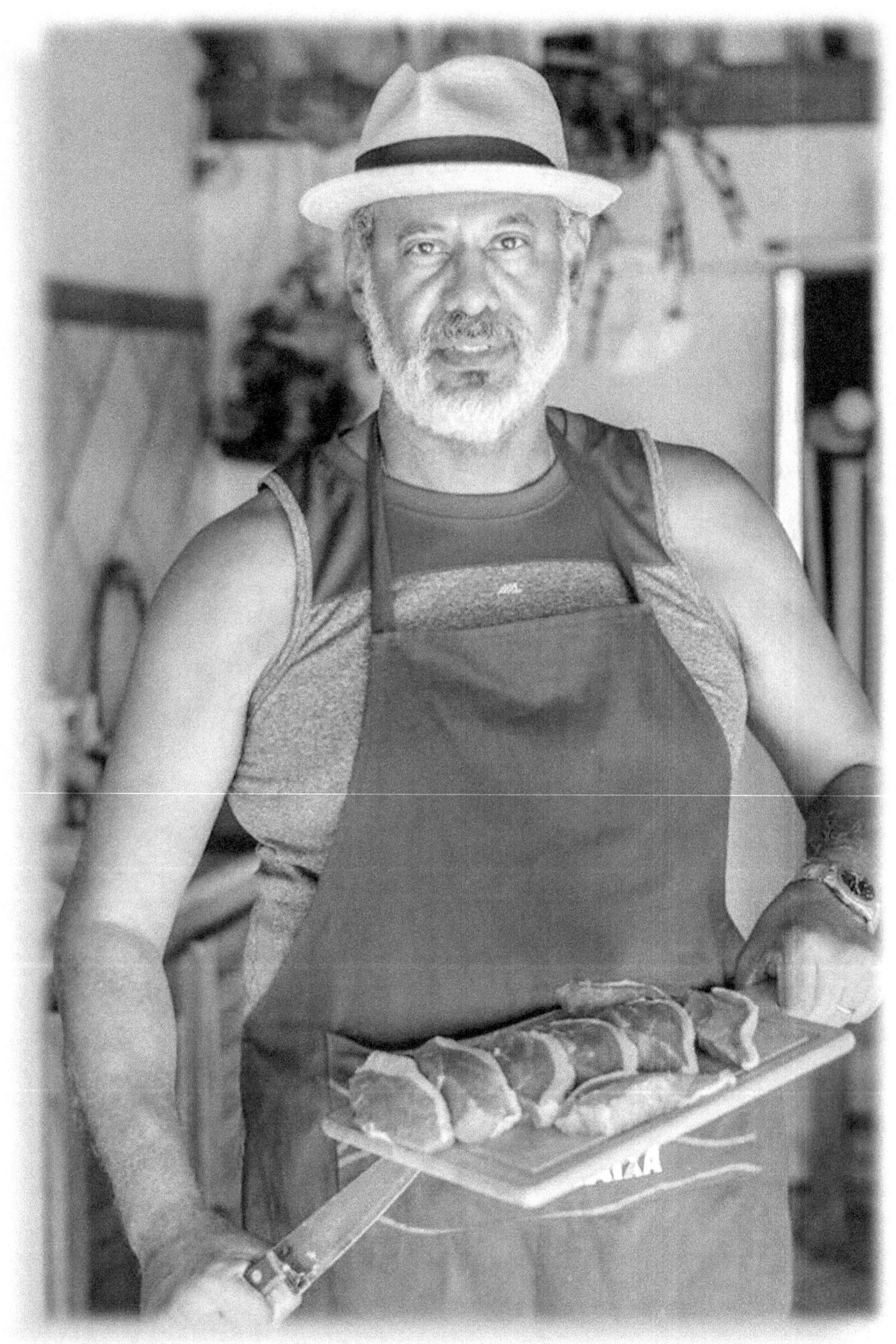

CHAPTER 1

INTRODUCTION TO THE CARNIVORE DIET

A dietary plan known as the "Carnivore Diet" has become very well-known in recent years. This eating style places a heavy emphasis on meat and only eats animal products. All plant-based foods are off limits for this diet, including grains, legumes, nuts, seeds, fruits, and vegetables. Eating solely animal products—such as beef, hog, chicken, fish, eggs, and dairy—is the main objective of the carnivore diet.

What is the Carnivore Diet?

The diet known as the "Carnivore Diet" is heavy in fat, low in carbohydrates, and high in protein. It is sometimes viewed as an extreme variant of the ketogenic diet or a stricter version of the Paleo diet. Advocates of the Carnivore Diet argue that it is a return to human nature, analogous to our hunter-gatherer predecessors' diet. They argue that by abandoning plant-based diets, people can achieve optimal health, reduce inflammation, and manage a range of chronic ailments.

The idea behind the diet is simple: consume solely animal products and stay away from anything plant-based. This means that organ meats, steaks, burgers, roasts, eggs, and high-fat dairy goods like cheese and butter are the usual mealtime fare. Some followers of the diet also include fish and seafood for variety and additional nutrients.

The History and Evolution of Carnivore Eating

The concept of carnivore eating is not new. Historically, many indigenous cultures and hunter-gatherer societies relied heavily on animal products for their sustenance, due to the scarcity of plant-based foods in their environments. Inuit populations, for example, subsisted primarily on a diet of fish, seal, whale, and other marine animals, with very few plant foods in their diet.

On the other hand, the contemporary Carnivore Diet is the result of a synthesis of current nutritional science and traditional dietary theories. It became well-known in the twenty-first century as part of the broader low-carb and ketogenic diet movements. The diet gained enormous popularity when social media emerged and people began sharing their success stories about how adopting a carnivorous lifestyle drastically improved their health, helped them lose weight, and enhanced their athletic ability.

Benefits and Potential Drawbacks

The Carnivore Diet boasts several potential benefits, as reported by its proponents:

Simplicity: The diet is straightforward and easy to follow, with no need to count calories or macronutrients.

Weight Loss: Many people experience rapid weight loss due to reduced appetite and the satiating effects of protein and fat.

Improved Digestion: The elimination of fibrous plant foods can lead to reduced bloating and digestive issues for some individuals.

Reduced Inflammation: A diet high in animal fats and proteins and low in carbohydrates may decrease inflammation markers in the body.

Mental Clarity: Some followers report enhanced mental clarity and focus, possibly due to stable blood sugar levels and ketosis.

Increased Energy: With the diet, you may avoid the energy dips that come with high-carb diets and have steady energy levels throughout the day.

However, the Carnivore Diet is not without its potential drawbacks and criticisms:

Nutritional Deficiencies: The exclusion of all plant-based foods raises concerns about deficiencies in certain vitamins, minerals, and phytonutrients.

Long-term Health Risks: The long-term health effects of an all-meat diet are poorly studied, and some experts are concerned about how it may affect cancer risk and heart health.

Environmental Impact: The high consumption of animal products raises ethical and environmental concerns related to animal welfare and sustainability.

Social Limitations: The restrictive nature of the diet can make social dining and eating out challenging.

Adaptation Period: Some individuals may experience initial side effects, such as fatigue, headaches, and digestive changes, as their bodies adjust to the diet.

The Carnivore Diet, which emphasizes a return to a more primitive style of eating, is a significant deviation from accepted dietary guidelines. Although the diet may be advantageous for some people, especially those who are trying to lose weight or find relief from a particular health issue, it is crucial to proceed cautiously and think about the diet's long-term effects on health and wellbeing. Before starting the Carnivore Diet, it is advised to speak with a healthcare provider as with any dietary adjustment.

CHAPTER 2:

UNDERSTANDING THE CARNIVORE DIET

The Carnivore Diet is a dietary approach that has accumulated both intrigue and skepticism in the nutritional world. Its focus solely on animal goods and total rejection of plant-based diets are its defining characteristics. This section attempts to compare this diet to other low-carb diets, dispel common misconceptions, and go deeper into the nutritional science underlying it.

Nutritional Science Behind Carnivore Eating

Fundamentally, the Carnivore Diet is based on the idea that an animal-based diet is more suitable for the physiology of humans. Proponents contend that without the anti-nutrients and inflammatory substances present in many plant-based meals, such a diet offers all the nutrients required for optimum health.

1. **Protein**: With all nine essential amino acids needed for muscle growth, repair, and general bodily function, animal products are complete protein sources. Consuming a lot of protein also increases satiety, which helps with weight management.

2. **Fat**: The diet is rich in saturated and monounsaturated fats, which are crucial for hormone production, brain health, and energy. Additionally, fat-soluble vitamins A, D, E, and K are carried by these lipids.

3. **Vitamins and Minerals**: Animal products are abundant in bioavailable nutrients, including vitamin B12, iron, zinc, and selenium. These nutrients are crucial for various bodily functions, including energy metabolism, immune response, and DNA synthesis.

4. **Absence of Carbohydrates**: Because the Carnivore Diet is almost entirely devoid of carbohydrates, it induces ketosis, a condition of altered metabolism. When the body is in ketosis, it burns fat as its main energy

source, which can lead to less inflammation, better blood sugar regulation, and weight loss.

Common Myths and Misconceptions

Despite its growing popularity, the Carnivore Diet is surrounded by several myths and misconceptions:

1. **Myth: It Causes Nutrient Deficiencies**: Opponents contend that vitamin and mineral shortages result from a diet deficient in plant-based foods. Advocates assert, however, that animal products offer all the elements required in more accessible forms.

2. **Myth: It's Unhealthy for the Heart**: Concerns about high saturated fat intake and its impact on heart health are common. Yet, recent studies challenge the direct link between saturated fat and cardiovascular disease.

3. **Myth: It's Bad for the Environment**: The environmental impact of a meat-centric diet is a point of contention. While industrial animal farming has significant environmental consequences, advocates of the diet often support sustainable and regenerative farming practices.

4. **Myth: It's Not Sustainable Long-Term**: Skeptics question the diet's sustainability, citing potential boredom and social challenges. However, many followers report high levels of satisfaction and adherence due to the simplicity and satiating nature of the diet.

Carnivore Diet vs. Other Low Carb Diets

The Carnivore Diet is often compared to other low-carb diets, such as the ketogenic and Paleo diets.

Here's how they differ:

1. **Ketogenic Diet**: Both diets cause ketosis, but the ketogenic diet allows for a greater range of foods, including low-carb veggies, nuts, and seeds. The Carnivore Diet is more restrictive and focuses solely on meals that come from animals.

2. **Paleo Diet**: The Paleo Diet emphasizes whole, unprocessed foods, including meat, fish, fruits, vegetables, nuts, and seeds. It excludes grains, legumes, and dairy. The Carnivore Diet takes this a step further by eliminating all plant-based foods.

3. **Atkins Diet**: The Atkins Diet is a low-carb eating plan that is phased in and begins with a tight induction period that is similar to the Carnivore Diet. But over time, it becomes less restrictive as carbohydrates are progressively added back in.

It is advisable to see a healthcare provider before beginning any new diet to be sure that the Carnivore Diet aligns with your unique health objectives and demands. The extreme Carnivore Diet is predicated on the idea that consuming a diet high in animal products is the most in line with human biology. Even if it might be advantageous for some, it's crucial to proceed cautiously and think through the long-term effects on sustainability and health.

CHAPTER 3:

THE ESSENTIALS OF THE CARNIVORE DIET

The main items and components of the diet, the significance of the type and source of meat, and the critical function of organ meats will all be covered in this part.

Key Foods and Ingredients

The foundation of the Carnivore Diet is built on a variety of animal products, each contributing unique nutritional benefits:

1. **Beef**: A staple of the diet, beef is a rich source of protein, iron, and B vitamins. It's preferred for its high nutrient density and satiety factor.

2. **Pork**: Another popular choice, pork provides a good mix of protein, fats, and micronutrients like thiamine and selenium.

3. **Chicken**: While leaner than red meats, chicken is a versatile protein source, often consumed for its affordability and ease of preparation.

4. **Fish and Seafood**: These are vital for their omega-3 fatty acids, which support heart and brain health. Salmon, mackerel, and sardines are particularly prized.

5. **Eggs**: Considered nature's multivitamin, eggs are a complete protein source and rich in choline, a nutrient essential for liver function and brain development.

6. **Dairy**: High-fat dairy products like cheese and butter are included for their calcium content and fat-soluble vitamins. However, some individuals may choose to limit dairy due to lactose intolerance or personal preference.

7. **Organ Meats**: Often referred to as "nature's superfoods," organ meats like liver, heart, and kidney are packed with nutrients, including vitamin A, iron, and coenzyme Q10.

Understanding Meat Quality and Sources

The quality of the meat is a critical consideration on the Carnivore Diet.

1. **Grass-Fed and Grass-Finished Beef**: Cattle that are grass-fed and finished tend to have higher levels of omega-3 fatty acids and conjugated linoleic acid (CLA), which are beneficial for health.

2. **Pasture-Raised Poultry and Pork**: Animals raised on pasture have a more natural diet and lifestyle, leading to meat that is potentially more nutrient-dense.

3. **Wild-Caught Fish**: Compared to farmed fish, wild-caught varieties generally have a better omega-3 to omega-6 fatty acid ratio, making them a healthier choice.

4. **Organic and Hormone-Free**: Opting for organic and hormone-free meats can reduce exposure to antibiotics, hormones, and pesticides, which may have adverse health effects.

Organ Meats and Their Importance

Offal, often known as organ meats, are the overlooked champions of the carnivore diet. They are rich in nutrients and offer a variety of vitamins and minerals.

1. **Liver**: Often considered the most nutrient-rich organ meat, liver is an excellent source of vitamin A, vitamin B12, iron, and folate.

2. **Heart**: Rich in CoQ10, an antioxidant that supports heart health and energy production, heart meat is also a good source of B vitamins and iron.

3. **Kidney**: High in selenium and B vitamins, kidney meat supports immune function and energy metabolism.

4. **Bone Marrow**: A delicacy in many cultures, bone marrow is rich in healthy fats, collagen, and nutrients like vitamin B12 and iron.

A wide range of nutrients can be ensured by including a variety of organ meats in the diet, which is particularly crucial when plant-based meals are scarce. They can be cooked in a variety of ways, such as pan-frying or creating nutrient-rich broths and pâtés.

A key feature of the carnivore diet is its concentration on animal products, particularly organ meats that are high in nutrients and of high quality. Anyone considering or adhering to this dietary plan must comprehend the main meals and ingredients as well as the significance of getting premium meats. As with any diet, it's critical to pay attention to your body's signals and adjust as necessary to maintain your best possible health and wellbeing.

CHAPTER 4

THE RULES OF CARNIVORE EATING

The simplicity of the Carnivore Diet, which only includes animal products, is what sets it apart. Nonetheless, there are several rules in this framework to guarantee the best possible nutrition and health results. Here, we'll go over the ins and outs of the Carnivore Diet, go into detail on what macro- and micronutrients are, and talk about how important electrolyte balance and hydration are.

Do's and Don'ts of the Carnivore Diet

To successfully adhere to the Carnivore Diet, it's important to understand the fundamental rules:

Do's:

1. **Prioritize Meat**: Meat, especially ruminant meat (beef, lamb, and bison) because of its high nutrient density, is the mainstay of the diet.

2. **Include a Variety of Animal Products**: Incorporate a range of animal foods, including poultry, pork, fish, eggs, and dairy (if tolerated), to ensure a broad spectrum of nutrients.

3. **Emphasize Organ Meats**: Consume organ meats regularly for their unparalleled nutrient content, including vitamins A, B12, and iron.

4. **Stay Hydrated**: Drink plenty of water throughout the day to maintain hydration levels.

5. **Monitor Electrolyte Intake**: Make sure you are getting enough electrolytes, especially the sodium, potassium, and magnesium that are contained in animal foods and can be added as supplements if needed.

Don'ts:

1. **Avoid Plant-Based Foods**: This includes fruits, vegetables, grains, legumes, nuts, and seeds, which are excluded from the diet.

2. **Limit Processed Meats**: While some processed meats can be included, it's best to limit them due to potential additives and lower nutrient quality.

3. **Steer Clear of Sugars and Sweeteners**: All forms of sugar and artificial sweeteners are to be avoided.

4. **Avoid Vegetable Oils**: Stick to animal fats for cooking and avoid vegetable oils, which are not permitted on the diet.

5. **Be Cautious with Dairy**: Because they are sensitive to dairy proteins or have a lactose intolerance, some people may need to limit or avoid dairy products.

Understanding Macros and Micros

The macronutrient makeup of the carnivore diet is distinct since it emphasizes fat and protein while consuming little in the way of carbs.

1. **Protein**: The diet is high in protein, which is essential for muscle repair, hormone production, and overall bodily functions. Aim for a moderate protein intake, balancing it with fat for energy.

2. **Fat**: Animal fats are a primary energy source on the Carnivore Diet. They provide essential fatty acids and help with the absorption of fat-soluble vitamins.

3. **Carbohydrates**: Since the diet excludes plant-based foods, carbohydrate intake is minimal. This can lead to a state of ketosis, where the body burns fat for fuel instead of carbohydrates.

Micronutrients are also crucial, and the Carnivore Diet provides many vitamins and minerals through organ meats, seafood, and other animal products. However, it's important to be mindful of potential nutrient gaps, such as vitamin C and fiber, and adjust the diet accordingly.

Hydration and Electrolyte Balance

On any diet, but especially the Carnivore Diet, where the body could experience major metabolic alterations, hydration is essential. On any diet, but especially the Carnivore Diet, where the body could experience major metabolic alterations, hydration is essential:

1. **Water**: Adequate water intake is essential to support bodily functions, aid digestion, and prevent dehydration.

2. **Electrolytes**: The diet can lead to changes in electrolyte balance, especially during the initial adaptation phase. It's important to ensure sufficient intake of sodium, potassium, and magnesium to maintain electrolyte balance and prevent symptoms like fatigue and muscle cramps.

3. **Bone Broth**: Consuming bone broth is a natural way to replenish electrolytes while also providing collagen and other beneficial nutrients.

Anyone starting this nutritional path needs to be aware of the dos and don'ts, the significance of macronutrients and micronutrients, and the necessity of electrolyte balance and hydration. Individual reactions may differ as with any dietary strategy, so it's critical to pay attention to your body and modify as necessary for optimum health and wellbeing.

CHAPTER 5:

GETTING STARTED WITH THE CARNIVORE DIET

A few preparations and changes to your kitchen and eating habits are necessary before you start the Carnivore Diet. Setting up your carnivore kitchen, making a grocery list and stocking your pantry with necessary items, and making the sustainable and health-conscious switch to a carnivorous diet are all covered in this section.

Setting Up Your Carnivore Kitchen

The first step in your journey is to create an environment that supports carnivore eating.

Here are some tips to get started:

1. **Equip Your Kitchen**: Make sure you have all the equipment you'll need to prepare meat, including a grill or barbecue, a cast-iron skillet, a meat thermometer, and a decent pair of knives.

2. **Organize Your Space**: For convenience and to preserve freshness, allocate specific areas of your freezer and refrigerator to various kinds of meat and animal products.

3. **Stock Up on Cooking Fats**: Animal fats like tallow, lard, and ghee are ideal for cooking on the Carnivore Diet. Keep a supply of these fats on hand for frying, sautéing, and roasting.

Shopping List and Pantry Essentials

A well-planned grocery list is essential to a successful carnivorous diet.

The following are a few necessities to have:

1. **Meats**: Beef, pork, lamb, chicken, and turkey are all excellent protein sources. opt for a variety of cuts, including steaks, roasts, ground meat, and ribs.

2. **Organ Meats**: Liver, heart, kidney, and other organ meats are nutrient-dense and should be incorporated regularly into your diet.

3. **Seafood**: Salmon, mackerel, sardines, shrimp, and oysters provide essential omega-3 fatty acids and other vital nutrients.

4. **Eggs**: A staple on the Carnivore Diet, eggs are a versatile and nutrient-rich food.

5. **Dairy**: If tolerated, include high-fat dairy products like cheese, butter, and heavy cream.

6. **Bone Broth**: Homemade or store-bought bone broth is a great source of collagen, electrolytes, and hydration.

7. **Seasonings**: While spices and herbs are technically plant-based, small amounts can be used for flavoring. Prioritize salt for electrolyte balance and taste enhancement.

Transitioning to a Carnivore Diet

Making the switch to a carnivore diet can be a significant change for your body.

Here are some steps to ease the transition:

1. **Start Gradually**: If you're currently eating a standard diet, begin by reducing your intake of carbohydrates and increasing your consumption of animal products over a few weeks.

2. **Listen to Your Body**: Pay attention to how your body responds to the dietary change. Adjust your fat and protein intake based on your energy levels, hunger, and overall well-being.

3. **Stay Hydrated**: Drink plenty of water to support your body's adjustment to a higher protein and fat intake.

4. **Monitor Electrolytes**: As your body adapts to the diet, you may experience shifts in electrolyte balance. Ensure adequate intake of sodium, potassium, and magnesium to prevent symptoms like fatigue or muscle cramps.

5. **Expect an Adaptation Period**: It's common to experience a transition period, often referred to as the "keto flu," as your body adapts to using fat for fuel instead of carbohydrates. Symptoms like headaches, fatigue, and irritability are temporary and should subside within a few weeks.

6. **Focus on Quality**: Prioritize high-quality, grass-fed, and pasture-raised meats and wild-caught seafood to maximize the nutritional benefits of the diet.

7. **Be Prepared for Social Situations**: Eating a carnivore diet can be challenging in social settings. Plan ahead by bringing your own food to events or choosing restaurants that offer suitable options.

8. **Seek Support**: Joining online communities or finding local groups of like-minded individuals can provide support, encouragement, and tips for navigating the carnivore lifestyle.

Setting up your kitchen, making a shopping list of necessary items, and implementing the diet gradually are the first steps in starting the Carnivore Diet. You can start a carnivorous journey that promotes your health and wellb.eing by concentrating on high-quality animal products and paying attention to your body's needs. It's crucial to speak with a healthcare provider before making any dietary changes to be sure the plan is suitable for your unique needs and objectives.

CHAPTER 6:

CARNIVORE DIET RECIPES: BREAKFAST

These delicious carnivore breakfast recipes will take you on an adventure in cooking. Simpleness and nutrition are the main priorities while creating each recipe, so you can look forward to a fulfilling start to the day.

CLASSIC STEAK AND EGGS

Ingredients: 6 oz rib, eye steak, 2 large eggs, salt, and pepper.

Prep Time: 5 minutes

Cook Time: 10 minutes

Directions:

- ✓ Season the steak with salt and pepper.
- ✓ In a skillet, cook the steak to your desired doneness.
- ✓ Remove and let it rest. In the same pan, fry the eggs to your liking.
- ✓ Serve the steak sliced with eggs on the side.

Nutritional Information: Calories: 470, Protein: 48g, Fat: 30g

BACON-WRAPPED ASPARAGUS

Ingredients: 8 asparagus spears, 8 slices of bacon.

Prep Time: 5 minutes

Cook Time: 20 minutes

Directions:

✓ Wrap each asparagus spear with a slice of bacon.
✓ Place on a baking sheet and bake at 400°F for 20 minutes, or until bacon is crispy.

Nutritional Information: Calories: 240, Protein: 15g, Fat: 20g

SMOKED SALMON OMELETS

Ingredients: 3 eggs, 2 oz smoked salmon, 1 tbsp butter, salt, and pepper.

Prep Time: 5 minutes

Cook Time: 5 minutes

Directions:

✓ Beat the eggs with salt and pepper.
✓ In a skillet, melt the butter and pour in the eggs.
✓ Cook until almost set, then add smoked salmon.
✓ Fold the omelet and serve.

Nutritional Information: Calories: 320, Protein: 27g, Fat: 22g

PORK BELLY BITES

Ingredients: 1 lb. pork belly, salt, and pepper.

Prep Time: 5 minutes

Cook Time: 1 hour

Directions:

✓ Cut the pork belly into bite-sized pieces.

✓ Season with salt and pepper.
✓ Roast at 400°F for 1 hour, or until crispy.

Nutritional Information: Calories: 580, Protein: 11g, Fat: 58g

BEEF LIVER PÂTÉ

Ingredients: 1 lb. beef liver, 1/4 cup butter, 1 onion, salt, and pepper.

Prep Time: 10 minutes

Cook Time: 15 minutes

Directions:

✓ Sauté the onion in butter until translucent.
✓ Add the liver and cook until browned.
✓ Blend the liver and onions in a food processor until smooth.
✓ Season with salt and pepper.

Nutritional Information: Calories: 400, Protein: 27g, Fat: 30g

EGG MUFFINS

Ingredients: 6 eggs, 1/2 cup diced ham, salt, and pepper.

Prep Time: 5 minutes

Cook Time: 20 minutes

Directions:

✓ Whisk the eggs with salt and pepper.
✓ Stir in the diced ham.

✓ Pour the mixture into muffin tins and bake at 350°F for 20 minutes.

Nutritional Information: Calories: 140, Protein: 12g, Fat: 9g

SAUSAGE PATTIES

Ingredients: 1 lb. ground pork, 1 tsp salt, 1/2 tsp black pepper, 1/2 tsp sage.

Prep Time: 5 minutes

Cook Time: 10 minutes

Directions:

- ✓ Mix the ground pork with the seasonings.
- ✓ Form into patties and fry in a skillet over medium heat until cooked through.

Nutritional Information: Calories: 290, Protein: 20g, Fat: 23g

CHICKEN LIVER SCRAMBLE

Ingredients: 1/2 lb. chicken liver, 4 eggs, 1 tbsp butter, salt, and pepper.

Prep Time: 5 minutes

Cook Time: 10 minutes

Directions:

- ✓ In a skillet, melt the butter and add the chicken liver.
- ✓ Cook until browned. Beat the eggs and pour them over the liver. Scramble until the eggs are set.

Nutritional Information: Calories: 360, Protein: 33g, Fat: 22g

BONE MARROW BUTTER SPREAD

Ingredients: 2 beef marrow bones, 1/4 cup butter, salt.

Prep Time: 5 minutes

Cook Time: 15 minutes

Directions:

- ✓ Roast the marrow bones at 450°F for 15 minutes.
- ✓ Scoop out the marrow and mix with softened butter and salt.
- ✓ Spread on your favorite carnivore-approved bread or eat alone.

Nutritional Information: Calories: 210, Protein: 1g, Fat: 23g

CARNIVORE QUICHE

Ingredients: 6 eggs, 1/2 cup heavy cream, 1 cup diced bacon, salt, and pepper.

Prep Time: 10 minutes

Cook Time: 35 minutes

Directions:

- ✓ Whisk together eggs, heavy cream, salt, and pepper.
- ✓ Stir in the diced bacon.
- ✓ Pour into a pie dish and bake at 350°F for 35 minutes.

Nutritional Information: Calories: 280, Protein: 16g, Fat: 23g

All of these recipes follow the Carnivore Diet guidelines and offer a range of flavors and textures, all while giving you a nutrient-dense start to your day. Savor discovering these delicious carnivore foods as you start your nutritional journey.

CHAPTER 7

CARNIVORE DIET RECIPES: LUNCH

Try these delicious and filling carnivorous lunch ideas to liven up your midday meals. Simple, delicious, and nutritionally sound cooking techniques are used to create each dish, making for a satisfying and satisfying meal.

GRILLED RIB EYE STEAK

Ingredients: 1 lb. rib, eye steak, salt, and pepper.

Prep Time: 5 minutes

Cook Time: 10 minutes

Directions:

- ✓ Season the steak with salt and pepper.
- ✓ Grill over high heat for 5 minutes per side for medium-rare.
- ✓ Let it rest before slicing.

Nutritional Information: Calories: 670, Protein: 69g, Fat: 42g

BACON-WRAPPED CHICKEN THIGHS

Ingredients: 4 chicken thighs, 8 slices of bacon, salt, and pepper.

Prep Time: 10 minutes

Cook Time: 30 minutes

Directions:

- ✓ Wrap each chicken thigh with two slices of bacon.
- ✓ Season with salt and pepper.
- ✓ Bake at 400°F for 30 minutes, or until the chicken is cooked through.

Nutritional Information: Calories: 480, Protein: 38g, Fat: 34g

SEARED SALMON WITH LEMON BUTTER

Ingredients: 2 salmon fillets, 2 tbsp butter, 1 lemon, salt, and pepper.

Prep Time: 5 minutes

Cook Time: 10 minutes

Directions:

- ✓ Season the salmon with salt and pepper.
- ✓ In a skillet, melt the butter and add the salmon, skin-side down.
- ✓ Cook for 5 minutes, then flip and cook for another 2-3 minutes.
- ✓ Squeeze lemon juice over the top before serving.

Nutritional Information: Calories: 400, Protein: 34g, Fat: 28g

PORK CHOPS WITH CREAMY MUSHROOM SAUCE

Ingredients: 2 pork chops, 1 cup heavy cream, 1 cup sliced mushrooms, salt, and pepper.

Prep Time: 5 minutes

Cook Time: 20 minutes

Directions:

- ✓ Season the pork chops and sear in a skillet.
- ✓ Remove and set aside.
- ✓ In the same skillet, add mushrooms and cook until browned.
- ✓ Add heavy cream and simmer until thickened.
- ✓ Return the pork chops to the pan and coat with the sauce.

Nutritional Information: Calories: 550, Protein: 38g, Fat: 42g

BEEF AND EGG STIR-FRY

Ingredients: 1 lb. ground beef, 4 eggs, salt, and pepper.

Prep Time: 5 minutes

Cook Time: 10 minutes

Directions:

- ✓ Brown the ground beef in a skillet.
- ✓ Push the beef to one side and scramble the eggs on the other side.
- ✓ Mix together and season with salt and pepper.

Nutritional Information: Calories: 480, Protein: 46g, Fat: 30g

LAMB KEBABS

Ingredients: 1 lb. lamb cubes, salt, and pepper.

Prep Time: 5 minutes

Cook Time: 10 minutes

Directions:

- ✓ Season the lamb cubes with salt and pepper.
- ✓ Thread onto skewers and grill over medium heat until cooked to your liking.

Nutritional Information: Calories: 400, Protein: 38g, Fat: 26g

CHICKEN LIVER SALAD

Ingredients: 1/2 lb. chicken livers, 2 hard-boiled eggs, salt, and pepper.

Prep Time: 5 minutes

Cook Time: 10 minutes

Directions:

- ✓ Sauté the chicken livers in a skillet until cooked through.
- ✓ Slice the hard-boiled eggs.
- ✓ Arrange the livers and eggs on a plate and season with salt and pepper.

Nutritional Information: Calories: 300, Protein: 27g, Fat: 20g

BISON BURGERS

Ingredients: 1 lb. ground bison, salt, and pepper.

Prep Time: 5 minutes

Cook Time: 10 minutes

Directions:

- ✓ Form the ground bison into patties.
- ✓ Season with salt and pepper.

✓ Grill or pan-fry until cooked to your desired doneness.

Nutritional Information: Calories: 240, Protein: 28g, Fat: 14g

DUCK BREAST WITH ORANGE GLAZE

Ingredients: 2 duck breasts, 1/4 cup orange juice (optional), salt, and pepper.

Prep Time: 5 minutes

Cook Time: 15 minutes

Directions:

- ✓ Score the duck skin and season with salt and pepper.
- ✓ Sear skin-side down until crispy.
- ✓ Flip and cook until medium-rare.
- ✓ Deglaze the pan with orange juice and reduce to a glaze.
- ✓ Pour over the duck before serving.

Nutritional Information: Calories: 360, Protein: 34g, Fat: 22g

VENISON STEW

Ingredients: 1 lb. venison cubes, 2 cups beef broth, salt, and pepper.

Prep Time: 10 minutes

Cook Time: 2 hours

Directions:

- ✓ Brown the venison in a pot.
- ✓ Add beef broth and season with salt and pepper.

✓ Simmer on low heat for 2 hours, or until the venison is tender.

Nutritional Information: Calories: 300, Protein: 52g, Fat: 8g

TURKEY DRUMSTICKS

Ingredients: 2 turkey drumsticks, salt, and pepper.

Prep Time: 5 minutes

Cook Time: 1 hour

Directions:

✓ Season the drumsticks with salt and pepper.
✓ Roast at 375°F for 1 hour, or until cooked through.

Nutritional Information: Calories: 410, Protein: 58g, Fat: 18g

GRILLED SWORDFISH

Ingredients: 2 swordfish steaks, salt, and pepper.

Prep Time: 5 minutes

Cook Time: 10 minutes

Directions:

✓ Season the swordfish with salt and pepper.
✓ Grill over high heat for 5 minutes per side, or until cooked through.

Nutritional Information: Calories: 370, Protein: 39g, Fat: 21g

ROAST QUAIL

Ingredients: 4 quails, salt, and pepper.

Prep Time: 5 minutes

Cook Time: 25 minutes

Directions:

- ✓ Season the quails with salt and pepper.
- ✓ Roast at 400°F for 25 minutes, or until cooked through.

Nutritional Information: Calories: 340, Protein: 52g, Fat: 14g

BEEF HEART SKEWERS

Ingredients: 1 lb. beef heart, salt, and pepper.

Prep Time: 10 minutes

Cook Time: 10 minutes

Directions:

- ✓ Cut the beef heart into cubes and season with salt and pepper.
- ✓ Thread onto skewers and grill over medium heat until cooked to your liking.

Nutritional Information: Calories: 250, Protein: 38g, Fat: 8g

CRAB CAKES

Ingredients: 1 lb. crab meat, 1 egg, salt, and pepper.

Prep Time: 10 minutes

Cook Time: 10 minutes

Directions:

- ✓ Mix the crab meat with the egg, salt, and pepper.
- ✓ Form into patties and pan-fry until golden brown on both sides.

Nutritional Information: Calories: 160, Protein: 32g, Fat: 2g

CHAPTER 8

CARNIVORE DIET RECIPES: DINNER

These delicious carnivorous supper ideas will elevate your evening meals. All of the recipes are created to please your palate while following the requirements of the carnivore diet, meaning that your meals will be filling and full of nutrients.

HERB-CRUSTED RACK OF LAMB

Ingredients: 1 rack of lamb, 2 tbsp fresh rosemary, 2 tbsp fresh thyme, salt, and pepper.

Prep Time: 10 minutes

Cook Time: 25 minutes

Directions:

- ✓ Preheat your oven to 400°F.
- ✓ Season the rack of lamb with salt and pepper.
- ✓ Mix the chopped rosemary and thyme, and press onto the lamb.
- ✓ Roast for 25 minutes for medium-rare. Let it rest before slicing.

Nutritional Information: Calories: 330, Protein: 25g, Fat: 24g

BEEF TENDERLOIN WITH GORGONZOLA SAUCE

Ingredients: 1 lb. beef tenderloin, 1/2 cup gorgonzola cheese, 1/4 cup heavy cream, salt, and pepper.

Prep Time: 5 minutes

Cook Time: 20 minutes

Directions:

- ✓ Season the beef tenderloin with salt and pepper.
- ✓ Sear on all sides in a hot skillet, then transfer to the oven and roast at 400°F until desired doneness.
- ✓ For the sauce, melt the gorgonzola cheese in heavy cream over low heat until smooth.
- ✓ Pour over the sliced tenderloin.

Nutritional Information: Calories: 510, Protein: 42g, Fat: 36g

GARLIC BUTTER SCALLOPS

Ingredients: 1 lb. scallops, 4 tbsp butter, 2 cloves garlic, minced, salt, and pepper.

Prep Time: 5 minutes

Cook Time: 10 minutes

Directions:

- ✓ In a skillet, melt the butter over medium heat.
- ✓ Add the minced garlic and cook until fragrant.
- ✓ Add the scallops and sear for 2-3 minutes on each side.
- ✓ Season with salt and pepper.

Nutritional Information: Calories: 300, Protein: 24g, Fat: 22g

BACON-WRAPPED FILET MIGNON

Ingredients: 2 filet mignon steaks, 4 slices of bacon, salt, and pepper.

Prep Time: 5 minutes

Cook Time: 15 minutes

Directions:

- ✓ Wrap each steak with two slices of bacon and secure with toothpicks.
- ✓ Season with salt and pepper.
- ✓ Grill or pan-sear to your desired doneness.

Nutritional Information: Calories: 400, Protein: 36g, Fat: 28g

ROASTED BONE MARROW

Ingredients: 4 beef marrow bones, salt, and pepper.

Prep Time: 5 minutes

Cook Time: 20 minutes

Directions:

- ✓ Preheat the oven to 450°F.
- ✓ Place the marrow bones on a baking sheet and roast for 20 minutes.
- ✓ Season with salt and pepper and serve.

Nutritional Information: Calories: 300, Protein: 7g, Fat: 28g

DUCK CONFIT

Ingredients: 4 duck legs, 4 cups duck fat, salt, and pepper.

Prep Time: 10 minutes

Cook Time: 3 hours

Directions:

✓ Season the duck legs with salt and pepper.
✓ Place in a deep baking dish and cover with duck fat.
✓ Bake at 300°F for 3 hours.
✓ The meat should be tender and easily pull away from the bone.

Nutritional Information: Calories: 520, Protein: 43g, Fat: 38g

GRILLED T-BONE STEAK

Ingredients: 1 T-bone steak, salt, and pepper.

Prep Time: 5 minutes

Cook Time: 10 minutes

Directions:

✓ Season the T-bone steak with salt and pepper.
✓ Grill over high heat for 5 minutes per side for medium-rare.

Nutritional Information: Calories: 450, Protein: 42g, Fat: 30g

PORK BELLY ROAST

Ingredients: 2 lbs. pork belly, salt, and pepper.

Prep Time: 5 minutes

Cook Time: 2 hours

Directions:

✓ Score the skin of the pork belly.
✓ Season with salt and pepper.

✓ Roast at 350°F for 2 hours, or until the skin is crispy and the meat is tender.

Nutritional Information: Calories: 580, Protein: 11g, Fat: 58g

BEEF SHORT RIBS

Ingredients: 2 lbs. beef short ribs, salt, and pepper.

Prep Time: 5 minutes

Cook Time: 3 hours

Directions:

✓ Season the short ribs with salt and pepper.
✓ Place in a baking dish and cover with foil.
✓ Bake at 300°F for 3 hours, or until the meat is fall-off-the-bone tender.

Nutritional Information: Calories: 500, Protein: 40g, Fat: 38g

LOBSTER TAIL WITH BUTTER SAUCE

Ingredients: 2 lobster tails, 4 tbsp butter, salt, and pepper.

Prep Time: 5 minutes

Cook Time: 10 minutes

Directions:

✓ Split the lobster tails in half and season with salt and pepper.
✓ Grill or broil for 5 minutes.
✓ In a saucepan, melt the butter and serve as a dipping sauce for the lobster.

Nutritional Information: Calories: 290, Protein: 24g, Fat: 22g

GRILLED VENISON STEAKS

Ingredients: 2 venison steaks, salt, and pepper.

Prep Time: 5 minutes

Cook Time: 10 minutes

Directions:

- ✓ Season the venison steaks with salt and pepper.
- ✓ Grill over high heat for 5 minutes per side for medium-rare.

Nutritional Information: Calories: 200, Protein: 38g, Fat: 3g

ROASTED QUAIL WITH HERBS

Ingredients: 4 quails, 2 tbsp fresh thyme, 2 tbsp fresh rosemary, salt, and pepper.

Prep Time: 10 minutes

Cook Time: 25 minutes

Directions:

- ✓ Preheat the oven to 400°F.
- ✓ Stuff each quail with thyme and rosemary.
- ✓ Season with salt and pepper.
- ✓ Roast for 25 minutes, or until cooked through.

Nutritional Information: Calories: 340, Protein: 52g, Fat: 14g

BRAISED OXTAIL

Ingredients: 2 lbs. oxtail, 2 cups beef broth, salt, and pepper.

Prep Time: 10 minutes

Cook Time: 3 hours

Directions:

- ✓ Season the oxtail with salt and pepper.
- ✓ Brown in a pot, then add beef broth.
- ✓ Cover and simmer on low heat for 3 hours, or until the meat is tender.

Nutritional Information: Calories: 400, Protein: 40g, Fat: 26g

GRILLED SWORDFISH STEAKS

Ingredients: 2 swordfish steaks, salt, and pepper.

Prep Time: 5 minutes

Cook Time: 10 minutes

Directions:

- ✓ Season the swordfish steaks with salt and pepper.
- ✓ Grill over high heat for 5 minutes per side, or until cooked through.

Nutritional Information: Calories: 370, Protein: 39g, Fat: 21g

BEEF LIVER WITH ONIONS

Ingredients: 1 lb. beef liver, 1 onion, sliced, 2 tbsp butter, salt, and pepper.

Prep Time: 5 minutes

Cook Time: 15 minutes

Directions:

- ✓ In a skillet, melt the butter and sauté the sliced onion until caramelized.
- ✓ Remove the onions and set aside.
- ✓ In the same skillet, cook the liver until browned on both sides.
- ✓ Season with salt and pepper.
- ✓ Serve with the caramelized onions on top.

Nutritional Information: Calories: 320, Protein: 27g, Fat: 22g

These evening recipes are all delicious ways to round off the day, combining flavor and nutrition in a way that is consistent with the principles of the carnivore diet. Savor these delicious works of art while you satiate your cravings and nourishing your body.

CHAPTER 9:

CARNIVORE DIET RECIPES: SNACKS AND SIDES

Taste these delicious, diet-friendly carnivorous snacks and side dishes. Every meal is designed to fit with the meat-eating philosophy and work well as an accompaniment to your main courses or as a filling snack.

CRISPY PORK RINDS

Ingredients: Pork skin, salt.

Prep Time: 5 minutes

Cook Time: 2 hours

Directions:

- ✓ Cut the pork skin into small pieces.
- ✓ Bake at 200°F for 2 hours or until dry.
- ✓ Deep fry the dried pieces until puffy and crispy.
- ✓ Season with salt.

Nutritional Information: Calories: 80, Protein: 9g, Fat: 5g (per serving)

BACON-WRAPPED JALAPEÑO POPPERS

Ingredients: 6 jalapeños, 12 slices of bacon, 6 oz cream cheese.

Prep Time: 15 minutes

Cook Time: 20 minutes

Directions:

- ✓ Slice the jalapeños in half and remove the seeds.
- ✓ Fill each half with cream cheese and wrap with a slice of bacon.
- ✓ Bake at 400°F for 20 minutes.

Nutritional Information: Calories: 150, Protein: 5g, Fat: 14g (per popper)

BEEF JERKY

Ingredients: 1 lb. lean beef, salt, black pepper.

Prep Time: 10 minutes

Cook Time: 4 hours

Directions:

- ✓ Slice the beef thinly against the grain.
- ✓ Season with salt and pepper.
- ✓ Place on a baking rack and dry in the oven at 170°F for 4 hours.

Nutritional Information: Calories: 70, Protein: 11g, Fat: 2g (per ounce)

DEVILED EGGS

Ingredients: 6 eggs, 3 tbsp mayonnaise, 1 tsp mustard, salt, and pepper.

Prep Time: 10 minutes

Cook Time: 10 minutes

Directions:

- ✓ Hard boil the eggs, peel and halve them.

- ✓ Remove the yolks and mix with mayonnaise, mustard, salt, and pepper.
- ✓ Fill the egg whites with the yolk mixture.

Nutritional Information: Calories: 90, Protein: 6g, Fat: 7g (per egg half)

CHICKEN WINGS

Ingredients: 1 lb. chicken wings, salt, pepper.

Prep Time: 5 minutes

Cook Time: 45 minutes

Directions:

- ✓ Season the wings with salt and pepper.
- ✓ Bake at 400°F for 45 minutes, or until crispy.

Nutritional Information: Calories: 100, Protein: 9g, Fat: 7g (per wing)

BONE BROTH

Ingredients: 2 lbs. mixed beef bones, water, salt.

Prep Time: 10 minutes

Cook Time: 24 hours

Directions:

- ✓ Place the bones in a slow cooker.
- ✓ Add enough water to cover and season with salt.
- ✓ Cook on low for 24 hours. Strain the broth and serve.

Nutritional Information: Calories: 40, Protein: 5g, Fat: 3g (per cup)

CHEESE CRISPS

Ingredients: Cheddar cheese, sliced.

Prep Time: 5 minutes

Cook Time: 10 minutes

Directions:

- ✓ Place small piles of cheese on a baking sheet lined with parchment paper.
- ✓ Bake at 400°F for 10 minutes, or until crispy.

Nutritional Information: Calories: 110, Protein: 7g, Fat: 9g (per crisp)

SARDINE SALAD

Ingredients: 1 can sardines, 1 tbsp olive oil, 1 tsp lemon juice, salt, and pepper.

Prep Time: 5 minutes

Cook Time: 0 minutes

Directions:

- ✓ Drain the sardines and place them in a bowl.
- ✓ Mix with olive oil, lemon juice, salt, and pepper.

Nutritional Information: Calories: 190, Protein: 23g, Fat: 10g (per serving)

PROSCIUTTO-WRAPPED ASPARAGUS

Ingredients: 12 asparagus spears, 12 slices prosciutto.

Prep Time: 10 minutes

Cook Time: 15 minutes

Directions:

- ✓ Wrap each asparagus spear with a slice of prosciutto.
- ✓ Bake at 400°F for 15 minutes.

Nutritional Information: Calories: 60, Protein: 5g, Fat: 4g (per wrapped spear)

BEEF BONE MARROW

Ingredients: 4 beef marrow bones, salt.

Prep Time: 5 minutes

Cook Time: 20 minutes

Directions:

- ✓ Place the marrow bones on a baking sheet.
- ✓ Roast at 450°F for 20 minutes.
- ✓ Season with salt and scoop out the marrow to eat.

Nutritional Information: Calories: 250, Protein: 1g, Fat: 27g (per bone)

LIVER PÂTÉ

Ingredients: 1 lb. chicken liver, 1/2 cup butter, 1 onion, salt, and pepper.

Prep Time: 10 minutes

Cook Time: 20 minutes

Directions:

- ✓ Sauté the onion in butter until translucent.
- ✓ Add the liver and cook until browned.
- ✓ Blend the liver and onions in a food processor until smooth.
- ✓ Season with salt and pepper.

Nutritional Information: Calories: 200, Protein: 14g, Fat: 15g (per serving)

BACON AND EGG CUPS

Ingredients: 6 slices of bacon, 6 eggs, salt, and pepper.

Prep Time: 5 minutes

Cook Time: 15 minutes

Directions:

- ✓ Line muffin tins with bacon slices.
- ✓ Crack an egg into each tin.
- ✓ Bake at 350°F for 15 minutes, or until the eggs are set.

Nutritional Information: Calories: 120, Protein: 9g, Fat: 9g (per cup)

SMOKED SALMON ROLL-UPS

Ingredients: 4 oz smoked salmon, 2 oz cream cheese.

Prep Time: 5 minutes

Cook Time: 0 minutes

Directions:

- ✓ Spread cream cheese on slices of smoked salmon.

✓ Roll up and cut into bite-sized pieces.

Nutritional Information: Calories: 100, Protein: 8g, Fat: 7g (per serving)

PORK BELLY STRIPS

Ingredients: 1 lb. pork belly, salt, and pepper.

Prep Time: 5 minutes

Cook Time: 1 hour

Directions:

- ✓ Cut the pork belly into strips.
- ✓ Season with salt and pepper.
- ✓ Roast at 400°F for 1 hour, or until crispy.

Nutritional Information: Calories: 520, Protein: 11g, Fat: 52g (per serving)

GRILLED SHRIMP SKEWERS

Ingredients: 1 lb. shrimp, salt, and pepper.

Prep Time: 10 minutes

Cook Time: 5 minutes

Directions:

- ✓ Season the shrimp with salt and pepper.
- ✓ Thread onto skewers and grill over high heat for 2-3 minutes per side.

Nutritional Information: Calories: 120, Protein: 23g, Fat: 2g (per serving)

A testament to the flexibility and gratification that the carnivore diet can provide, each of these snacks and sides will satisfy your palate and help you stick to your diet. Either you're searching for a satisfying snack or a side dish to go with it, these dishes will not disappoint.

CHAPTER 10

CARNIVORE DIET RECIPES: ORGAN MEATS

Try out these carnivore diet recipes to learn about the nutritious powerhouse that is organ meats. Each entree is created to highlight the distinct tastes and health advantages of various organ meats, offering a gourmet experience that suits your nutritious aspirations.

PAN-SEARED BEEF LIVER WITH ONIONS

Ingredients: 1 lb. beef liver, 1 onion, 2 tbsp butter, salt, and pepper.

Prep Time: 10 minutes

Cook Time: 15 minutes

Directions:

- ✓ Slice the onion and sauté in butter until caramelized.
- ✓ Remove onions and set aside.
- ✓ Slice the liver into thin strips, season with salt and pepper, and sear in the same pan for 2-3 minutes per side.
- ✓ Serve with the caramelized onions.

Nutritional Information: Calories: 250, Protein: 27g, Fat: 12g (per serving)

GRILLED CHICKEN HEARTS

Ingredients: 1 lb. chicken hearts, 2 tbsp olive oil, salt, and pepper.

Prep Time: 5 minutes

Cook Time: 10 minutes

Directions:

- ✓ Toss chicken hearts with olive oil, salt, and pepper.
- ✓ Thread onto skewers and grill over medium heat for 5 minutes per side, or until cooked through.

Nutritional Information: Calories: 180, Protein: 26g, Fat: 8g (per serving)

BRAISED LAMB KIDNEYS

Ingredients: 1 lb. lamb kidneys, 1 cup beef broth, 1 tbsp butter, salt, and pepper.

Prep Time: 10 minutes

Cook Time: 1 hour

Directions:

- ✓ Halve the kidneys and remove the central core.
- ✓ Season with salt and pepper.
- ✓ In a pot, melt the butter and brown the kidneys.
- ✓ Add beef broth and simmer on low heat for 1 hour, or until tender.

Nutritional Information: Calories: 210, Protein: 29g, Fat: 9g (per serving)

FRIED PORK BRAIN

Ingredients: 1 lb. pork brain, 1 cup flour, 2 eggs, salt, and pepper.

Prep Time: 15 minutes

Cook Time: 10 minutes

Directions:

- ✓ Soak the pork brain in cold water for 2 hours.
- ✓ Drain and slice.
- ✓ Dip in beaten eggs, then coat with flour seasoned with salt and pepper.
- ✓ Fry in hot oil until golden brown.

Nutritional Information: Calories: 320, Protein: 14g, Fat: 26g (per serving)

BEEF HEART STEW

Ingredients: 1 lb. beef heart, 2 cups beef broth, 1 onion, 2 carrots, salt, and pepper.

Prep Time: 10 minutes

Cook Time: 2 hours

Directions:

- ✓ Cube the beef heart.
- ✓ In a pot, sauté the chopped onion and sliced carrots.
- ✓ Add the beef heart and beef broth.
- ✓ Season with salt and pepper.
- ✓ Simmer on low heat for 2 hours, or until the heart is tender.

Nutritional Information: Calories: 220, Protein: 28g, Fat: 10g (per serving)

SAUTÉED CHICKEN GIZZARDS

Ingredients: 1 lb. chicken gizzards, 2 tbsp butter, salt, and pepper.

Prep Time: 10 minutes

Cook Time: 45 minutes

Directions:

- ✓ Clean the gizzards and slice them thinly.
- ✓ In a skillet, melt the butter and sauté the gizzards over medium heat for 45 minutes, or until tender.
- ✓ Season with salt and pepper.

Nutritional Information: Calories: 200, Protein: 30g, Fat: 8g (per serving)

GRILLED BEEF TONGUE

Ingredients: 1 beef tongue, 2 tbsp olive oil, salt, and pepper.

Prep Time: 10 minutes

Cook Time: 3 hours

Directions:

- ✓ Boil the beef tongue in water for 3 hours, or until tender.
- ✓ Peel off the outer layer.
- ✓ Slice, season with salt and pepper, and grill for a few minutes on each side.

Nutritional Information: Calories: 250, Protein: 21g, Fat: 18g (per serving)

PAN-FRIED VEAL SWEETBREADS

Ingredients: 1 lb. veal sweetbreads, 1 cup flour, 2 tbsp butter, salt, and pepper.

Prep Time: 10 minutes

Cook Time: 15 minutes

Directions:

- ✓ Soak sweetbreads in cold water for 2 hours.

- ✓ Drain and pat dry.
- ✓ Coat in flour seasoned with salt and pepper.
- ✓ Fry in butter until golden brown.

Nutritional Information: Calories: 310, Protein: 20g, Fat: 22g (per serving)

BAKED PORK SPLEEN

Ingredients: 1 lb. pork spleen, 2 tbsp olive oil, salt, and pepper.

Prep Time: 5 minutes

Cook Time: 30 minutes

Directions:

- ✓ Clean the spleen and slice it.
- ✓ Toss with olive oil, salt, and pepper.
- ✓ Bake at 350°F for 30 minutes.

Nutritional Information: Calories: 210, Protein: 34g, Fat: 8g (per serving)

LIVER AND ONIONS

Ingredients: 1 lb. calf liver, 2 onions, 2 tbsp butter, salt, and pepper.

Prep Time: 10 minutes

Cook Time: 20 minutes

Directions:

- ✓ Slice the onions and sauté in butter until caramelized.
- ✓ Remove onions and set aside.

- ✓ Slice the liver and season with salt and pepper.
- ✓ Sear in the same pan for 3-4 minutes per side.
- ✓ Serve with the caramelized onions.

Nutritional Information: Calories: 260, Protein: 27g, Fat: 14g (per serving)

GRILLED MARROW BONES

Ingredients: 4 beef marrow bones, salt, and pepper.

Prep Time: 5 minutes

Cook Time: 15 minutes

Directions:

- ✓ Season the marrow bones with salt and pepper.
- ✓ Grill over medium heat for 15 minutes, or until the marrow is soft.
- ✓ Scoop out the marrow to eat.

Nutritional Information: Calories: 300, Protein: 7g, Fat: 28g (per bone)

BEEF KIDNEY PIE

Ingredients: 1 lb. beef kidney, 1 pie crust, 1 cup beef broth, salt, and pepper.

Prep Time: 15 minutes

Cook Time: 1 hour

Directions:

- ✓ Clean and cube the kidney.
- ✓ Place in a pie dish with beef broth.

- ✓ Season with salt and pepper.
- ✓ Cover with pie crust and bake at 350°F for 1 hour.

Nutritional Information: Calories: 420, Protein: 26g, Fat: 30g (per serving)

FRIED DUCK LIVER

Ingredients: 1 lb. duck liver, 2 tbsp butter, salt, and pepper.

Prep Time: 5 minutes

Cook Time: 10 minutes

Directions:

- ✓ Season the duck liver with salt and pepper.
- ✓ Fry in butter over medium heat for 5 minutes per side.

Nutritional Information: Calories: 320, Protein: 27g, Fat: 22g (per serving)

BRAISED HEART WITH VEGETABLES

Ingredients: 1 beef heart, 2 carrots, 2 celery stalks, 2 cups beef broth, salt, and pepper.

Prep Time: 15 minutes

Cook Time: 2 hours

Directions:

- ✓ Cube the beef heart.
- ✓ Sauté chopped carrots and celery in a pot.
- ✓ Add the heart and beef broth.

- ✓ Season with salt and pepper.
- ✓ Simmer on low heat for 2 hours, or until the heart is tender.

Nutritional Information: Calories: 220, Protein: 28g, Fat: 10g (per serving)

PAN-SEARED VEAL LIVER

Ingredients: 1 lb. veal liver, 2 tbsp butter, salt, and pepper.

Prep Time: 5 minutes

Cook Time: 10 minutes

Directions:

- ✓ Slice the veal liver.
- ✓ Season with salt and pepper.
- ✓ Sear in butter over high heat for 5 minutes per side.

Nutritional Information: Calories: 270, Protein: 27g, Fat: 16g (per serving)

Take advantage of the rich flavors and variety these recipes offer, as well as the health benefits that come with eating organ meats. Each recipe for organ meat offers a different approach to include nutrient-dense alternatives into your carnivorous diet.

CHAPTER 11

CARNIVORE DIET RECIPES: SEAFOOD

Probe the depths of flavor with these dishes that emphasize seafood. These recipes are ideal for novice cooks as well as seasoned ones since they showcase the inherent flavor and nutritional benefits of different kinds of fish.

GARLIC BUTTER SHRIMP

Ingredients: 1 lb. shrimp, 4 tbsp butter, 2 cloves garlic, minced, salt, and pepper.

Prep Time: 5 minutes

Cook Time: 10 minutes

Directions:

- ✓ Melt the butter in a skillet and add the minced garlic.
- ✓ Sauté for a minute, then add the shrimp.
- ✓ Cook until the shrimp are pink and opaque.
- ✓ Season with salt and pepper.

Nutritional Information: Calories: 240, Protein: 24g, Fat: 15g (per serving)

GRILLED SALMON STEAKS

Ingredients: 2 salmon steaks, 2 tbsp olive oil, salt, and pepper.

Prep Time: 5 minutes

Cook Time: 10 minutes

Directions:

- ✓ Brush the salmon steaks with olive oil and season with salt and pepper.
- ✓ Grill over medium heat for 5 minutes on each side, or until cooked through.

Nutritional Information: Calories: 370, Protein: 34g, Fat: 25g (per steak)

PAN-SEARED SCALLOPS

Ingredients: 1 lb. scallops, 2 tbsp butter, salt, and pepper.

Prep Time: 5 minutes

Cook Time: 5 minutes

Directions:

- ✓ Pat the scallops dry and season with salt and pepper.
- ✓ Heat the butter in a skillet over high heat.
- ✓ Add the scallops and sear for 2-3 minutes on each side.

Nutritional Information: Calories: 200, Protein: 21g, Fat: 11g (per serving)

BAKED COD WITH LEMON

Ingredients: 1 lb. cod fillets, 2 lemons, 2 tbsp olive oil, salt, and pepper.

Prep Time: 5 minutes

Cook Time: 15 minutes

Directions:

- ✓ Preheat the oven to 400°F.
- ✓ Place the cod fillets in a baking dish.

- ✓ Drizzle with olive oil and squeeze lemon juice over the top.
- ✓ Season with salt and pepper.
- ✓ Bake for 15 minutes, or until the fish flakes easily with a fork.

Nutritional Information: Calories: 190, Protein: 23g, Fat: 10g (per serving)

LOBSTER TAIL WITH BUTTER SAUCE

Ingredients: 2 lobster tails, 4 tbsp butter, salt, and pepper.

Prep Time: 5 minutes

Cook Time: 10 minutes

Directions:

- ✓ Cut the lobster tails down the middle and season with salt and pepper.
- ✓ Broil for 5 minutes.
- ✓ In a saucepan, melt the butter and pour over the cooked lobster tails.

Nutritional Information: Calories: 290, Protein: 24g, Fat: 22g (per tail)

GRILLED OCTOPUS

Ingredients: 1 lb. octopus, 2 tbsp olive oil, salt, and pepper.

Prep Time: 10 minutes

Cook Time: 20 minutes

Directions:

- ✓ Precook the octopus in boiling water for 15 minutes.
- ✓ Then, marinate with olive oil, salt, and pepper.

✓ Grill over high heat for 5 minutes on each side.

Nutritional Information: Calories: 170, Protein: 25g, Fat: 7g (per serving)

SEARED TUNA STEAKS

Ingredients: 2 tuna steaks, 2 tbsp sesame oil, salt, and pepper.

Prep Time: 5 minutes

Cook Time: 5 minutes

Directions:

✓ Brush the tuna steaks with sesame oil and season with salt and pepper.
✓ Sear in a hot skillet for 2-3 minutes on each side.

Nutritional Information: Calories: 220, Protein: 31g, Fat: 10g (per steak)

BAKED MACKEREL

Ingredients: 1 mackerel, 2 tbsp olive oil, salt, and pepper.

Prep Time: 5 minutes

Cook Time: 20 minutes

Directions:

✓ Preheat the oven to 375°F.
✓ Clean and gut the mackerel.
✓ Rub with olive oil and season with salt and pepper.
✓ Bake for 20 minutes, or until cooked through.

Nutritional Information: Calories: 310, Protein: 22g, Fat: 24g (per serving)

FRIED SARDINES

Ingredients: 1 lb. sardines, 2 tbsp olive oil, salt, and pepper.

Prep Time: 5 minutes

Cook Time: 5 minutes

Directions:

- ✓ Clean and gut the sardines.
- ✓ Heat the olive oil in a skillet and fry the sardines for 2-3 minutes on each side.
- ✓ Season with salt and pepper.

Nutritional Information: Calories: 220, Protein: 25g, Fat: 12g (per serving)

CRAYFISH BOIL

Ingredients: 2 lbs. crayfish, 4 tbsp seafood seasoning, salt.

Prep Time: 10 minutes

Cook Time: 15 minutes

Directions:

- ✓ Fill a large pot with water and add seafood seasoning and salt.
- ✓ Bring to a boil and add the crayfish.
- ✓ Cook for 15 minutes, or until the crayfish turn bright red.
- ✓ Drain and serve.

Nutritional Information: Calories: 90, Protein: 18g, Fat: 1g (per serving)

OYSTERS ON THE HALF SHELL

Ingredients: 12 oysters, lemon wedges.

Prep Time: 10 minutes

Cook Time: 0 minutes

Directions:

- ✓ Shuck the oysters and place them on a bed of ice.
- ✓ Serve with lemon wedges.

Nutritional Information: Calories: 10, Protein: 1g, Fat: 0g (per oyster)

GRILLED SWORDFISH WITH HERB BUTTER

Ingredients: 2 swordfish steaks, 4 tbsp butter, 1 tbsp mixed herbs (parsley, thyme, rosemary), salt, and pepper.

Prep Time: 5 minutes

Cook Time: 10 minutes

Directions:

- ✓ Season the swordfish steaks with salt and pepper.
- ✓ Grill over medium heat for 5 minutes on each side.
- ✓ Mix the butter with the herbs and melt over the cooked steaks.

Nutritional Information: Calories: 370, Protein: 34g, Fat: 25g (per steak)

CAVIAR ON SCRAMBLED EGGS

Ingredients: 4 eggs, 2 tbsp caviar, 2 tbsp butter, salt, and pepper.

Prep Time: 5 minutes

Cook Time: 5 minutes

Directions:

- ✓ Scramble the eggs in butter.
- ✓ Season with salt and pepper.
- ✓ Top with caviar before serving.

Nutritional Information: Calories: 180, Protein: 12g, Fat: 14g (per serving)

SMOKED SALMON ROLL-UPS

Ingredients: 4 oz smoked salmon, 2 oz cream cheese.

Prep Time: 5 minutes

Cook Time: 0 minutes

Directions:

- ✓ Spread cream cheese on slices of smoked salmon.
- ✓ Roll up and cut into bite-sized pieces.

Nutritional Information: Calories: 100, Protein: 8g, Fat: 7g (per serving)

CLAMS IN GARLIC BUTTER SAUCE

Ingredients: 2 lbs. clams, 4 tbsp butter, 2 cloves garlic, minced, salt, and pepper.

Prep Time: 10 minutes

Cook Time: 10 minutes

Directions:

- ✓ Melt the butter in a pot and add the minced garlic.
- ✓ Add the clams and cover.
- ✓ Cook until the clams open, about 10 minutes.
- ✓ Season with salt and pepper.

Nutritional Information: Calories: 200, Protein: 16g, Fat: 14g (per serving)

Through every phase of these seafood recipes serve up a tasty and different way that you can enjoy the abundance of the sea while following a carnivorous diet. These dishes will fulfill your appetites and supply vital nutrients, ranging from basic grilled fish to opulent caviar.

CHAPTER 12

CARNIVORE DIET RECIPES: BONE BROTHS AND SOUPS

Pamper your body with these robust and nutritious bone broth and soup recipes from the carnivore diet. Every dish is thoughtfully prepared to offer a nourishing and cozy experience that will appeal to both beginning users and dietary the experts.

BASIC BEEF BONE BROTH

Ingredients: 3 lbs. beef bones, 2 tbsp apple cider vinegar, water, salt.

Prep Time: 10 minutes

Cook Time: 24 hours

Directions:

- ✓ Place the beef bones in a large pot and cover with water.
- ✓ Add apple cider vinegar and let sit for 30 minutes.
- ✓ Bring to a boil, then reduce to a simmer.
- ✓ Simmer for 24 hours, skimming off any foam that forms.
- ✓ Season with salt to taste.
- ✓ Strain and store.

Nutritional Information: Calories: 40, Protein: 5g, Fat: 3g (per cup)

CHICKEN BONE BROTH

Ingredients: 1 whole chicken carcass, 2 tbsp apple cider vinegar, water, salt.

Prep Time: 10 minutes

Cook Time: 24 hours

Directions:

- ✓ Put the chicken carcass in a big pot and add water to cover it.
- ✓ After adding the apple cider vinegar, wait 30 minutes.
- ✓ After bringing to a boil, lower heat to a simmer.
- ✓ Skim any forming froth and simmer for a whole day.
- ✓ Add salt to taste to season. After straining, store.

Nutritional Information: Calories: 30, Protein: 4g, Fat: 2g (per cup)

FISH BONE BROTH

Ingredients: 2 lbs. fish bones, 2 tbsp apple cider vinegar, water, salt.

Prep Time: 10 minutes

Cook Time: 8 hours

Directions:

- ✓ Place the fish bones in a large pot and cover with water.
- ✓ Add apple cider vinegar and let sit for 30 minutes.
- ✓ Bring to a boil, then reduce to a simmer.
- ✓ Simmer for 8 hours, skimming off any foam that forms.
- ✓ Season with salt to taste. Strain and store.

Nutritional Information: Calories: 25, Protein: 4g, Fat: 1g (per cup)

PORK BONE BROTH

Ingredients: 3 lbs. pork bones, 2 tbsp apple cider vinegar, water, salt.

Prep Time: 10 minutes

Cook Time: 24 hours

Directions:

- ✓ Place the pork bones in a large pot and cover with water.
- ✓ Add apple cider vinegar and let sit for 30 minutes.
- ✓ Bring to a boil, then reduce to a simmer.
- ✓ Simmer for 24 hours, skimming off any foam that forms.
- ✓ Season with salt to taste. Strain and store.

Nutritional Information: Calories: 50, Protein: 6g, Fat: 3g (per cup)

BEEF MARROW BONE BROTH

Ingredients: 2 lbs. beef marrow bones, 2 tbsp apple cider vinegar, water, salt.

Prep Time: 10 minutes

Cook Time: 24 hours

Directions:

- ✓ Place the marrow bones in a large pot and cover with water.
- ✓ Add apple cider vinegar and let sit for 30 minutes.
- ✓ Bring to a boil, then reduce to a simmer.
- ✓ Simmer for 24 hours, skimming off any foam that forms.
- ✓ Season with salt to taste.
- ✓ Strain and store.

Nutritional Information: Calories: 60, Protein: 5g, Fat: 4g (per cup)

LAMB BONE BROTH

Ingredients: 3 lbs. lamb bones, 2 tbsp apple cider vinegar, water, salt.

Prep Time: 10 minutes

Cook Time: 24 hours

Directions:

- ✓ Place the lamb bones in a large pot and cover with water.
- ✓ Add apple cider vinegar and let sit for 30 minutes.
- ✓ Bring to a boil, then reduce to a simmer.
- ✓ Simmer for 24 hours, skimming off any foam that forms.
- ✓ Season with salt to taste.
- ✓ After straining, store.

Nutritional Information: Calories: 45, Protein: 6g, Fat: 3g (per cup)

TURKEY BONE BROTH

Ingredients: 1 whole turkey carcass, 2 tbsp apple cider vinegar, water, salt.

Prep Time: 10 minutes

Cook Time: 24 hours

Directions:

- ✓ Place the turkey carcass in a large pot and cover with water.
- ✓ Add apple cider vinegar and let sit for 30 minutes.
- ✓ Bring to a boil, then reduce to a simmer.
- ✓ Simmer for 24 hours, skimming off any foam that forms.
- ✓ Season with salt to taste.
- ✓ Pour through and store.

Nutritional Information: Calories: 35, Protein: 5g, Fat: 2g (per cup)

VENISON BONE BROTH

Ingredients: 3 lbs. venison bones, 2 tbsp apple cider vinegar, water, salt.

Prep Time: 10 minutes

Cook Time: 24 hours

Directions:

- ✓ Place the venison bones in a large pot and cover with water.
- ✓ Add apple cider vinegar and let sit for 30 minutes.
- ✓ Bring to a boil, then reduce to a simmer.
- ✓ Simmer for 24 hours, skimming off any foam that forms.
- ✓ Season with salt to taste.
- ✓ Strain and store.

Nutritional Information: Calories: 40, Protein: 6g, Fat: 2g (per cup)

DUCK BONE BROTH

Ingredients: 2 lbs. duck bones, 2 tbsp apple cider vinegar, water, salt.

Prep Time: 10 minutes

Cook Time: 24 hours

Directions:

- ✓ Place the duck bones in a large pot and cover with water.

- ✓ Add apple cider vinegar and let sit for 30 minutes.
- ✓ Bring to a boil, then reduce to a simmer.
- ✓ Simmer for 24 hours, skimming off any foam that forms.
- ✓ Season with salt to taste.
- ✓ Strain and store.

Nutritional Information: Calories: 35, Protein: 5g, Fat: 2g (per cup)

OXTAIL SOUP

Ingredients: 2 lbs. oxtail, 2 cups beef broth, salt, and pepper.

Prep Time: 10 minutes

Cook Time: 3 hours

Directions:

- ✓ Place the oxtail in a pot and cover with beef broth.
- ✓ Season with salt and pepper.
- ✓ Bring to a boil, then reduce to a simmer.
- ✓ Simmer for 3 hours, or until the meat is tender and falling off the bone.
- ✓ Strain and serve.

Nutritional Information: Calories: 220, Protein: 22g, Fat: 14g (per serving)

FISH HEAD SOUP

Ingredients: 2 fish heads, 2 cups fish broth, salt, and pepper.

Prep Time: 10 minutes

Cook Time: 1 hour

Directions:

- ✓ Place the fish heads in a pot and cover with fish broth.
- ✓ Season with salt and pepper.
- ✓ Bring to a boil, then reduce to a simmer.
- ✓ Simmer for 1 hour.
- ✓ Strain and serve.

Nutritional Information: Calories: 80, Protein: 12g, Fat: 3g (per serving)

CHICKEN HEART SOUP

Ingredients: 1 lb. chicken hearts, 2 cups chicken broth, salt, and pepper.

Prep Time: 10 minutes

Cook Time: 1 hour

Directions:

- ✓ Place the chicken hearts in a pot and cover with chicken broth.
- ✓ Season with salt and pepper.
- ✓ Bring to a boil, then reduce to a simmer.
- ✓ Simmer for 1 hour, or until the hearts are tender.
- ✓ Strain and serve.

Nutritional Information: Calories: 160, Protein: 26g, Fat: 5g (per serving)

BEEF TRIPE SOUP

Ingredients: 2 lbs. beef tripe, 2 cups beef broth, salt, and pepper.

Prep Time: 10 minutes

Cook Time: 3 hours

Directions:

- ✓ Clean the tripe and cut into bite-sized pieces.
- ✓ Place in a pot and cover with beef broth.
- ✓ Season with salt and pepper.
- ✓ Bring to a boil, then reduce to a simmer.
- ✓ Simmer for 3 hours, or until the tripe is tender.
- ✓ Strain and serve.

Nutritional Information: Calories: 180, Protein: 24g, Fat: 8g (per serving)

<u>PORK BONE SOUP</u>

Ingredients: 3 lbs. pork bones, 2 cups pork broth, salt, and pepper.

Prep Time: 10 minutes

Cook Time: 24 hours

Directions:

- ✓ Place the pork bones in a large pot and cover with pork broth.
- ✓ Season with salt and pepper.
- ✓ Bring to a boil, then reduce to a simmer.
- ✓ Simmer for 24 hours, skimming off any foam that forms.
- ✓ **Strain and serve.**

Nutritional Information: Calories: 50, Protein: 7g, Fat: 3g (per cup)

LAMB NECK SOUP

Ingredients: 2 lbs. lamb neck, 2 cups lamb broth, salt, and pepper.

Prep Time: 10 minutes

Cook Time: 3 hours

Directions:

- ✓ Place the lamb neck in a pot and cover with lamb broth.
- ✓ Season with salt and pepper.
- ✓ Bring to a boil, then reduce to a simmer.
- ✓ Simmer for 3 hours, or until the meat is tender and falling off the bone.
- ✓ Strain and serve.

Nutritional Information: Calories: 210, Protein: 22g, Fat: 12g (per serving)

For individuals who are on a carnivorous diet, these bone broths and soups provide a substantial and inviting choice. These recipes give a tasty way to include a range of meaty organs and bones in your diet, the fact that you're searching for a simple broth to sip on or a hearty soup to enjoy as a meal.

CHAPTER 13

CARNIVORE DIET RECIPES: SAUCES AND CONDIMENTS

These appealing, simple-to-make sauces and seasonings can enhance your meat recipes. Many of the recipes are designed to fit within the carnivore diet directives, but they may also be used to enhance your meat-heavy meals.

CLASSIC BONE MARROW BUTTER

Ingredients: 4 beef marrow bones, 1/2 cup butter, salt.

Prep Time: 5 minutes

Cook Time: 15 minutes

Directions:

- ✓ Roast the marrow bones at 450°F for 15 minutes.
- ✓ Scoop out the marrow and mix with softened butter and salt.
- ✓ Use as a spread or to top steaks.

Nutritional Information: Calories: 100, Protein: 1g, Fat: 11g (per tablespoon)

BEEF TALLOW MAYO

Ingredients: 1 egg yolk, 1 cup beef tallow (melted), 1 tsp lemon juice, salt.

Prep Time: 10 minutes

Cook Time: 0 minutes

Directions:

✓ Whisk the egg yolk with lemon juice and salt.
✓ Slowly drizzle in the melted tallow, whisking continuously until emulsified.

Nutritional Information: Calories: 100, Protein: 0g, Fat: 11g (per tablespoon)

CREAMY HORSERADISH SAUCE

Ingredients: 1/2 cup sour cream, 2 tbsp prepared horseradish, salt.

Prep Time: 5 minutes

Cook Time: 0 minutes

Directions:

✓ Mix the sour cream with horseradish and salt.
✓ Adjust the amount of horseradish to your taste.
✓ Serve with beef.

Nutritional Information: Calories: 60, Protein: 1g, Fat: 6g (per tablespoon)

CARNIVORE GRAVY

Ingredients: 2 cups beef broth, 1/4 cup beef drippings, salt, and pepper.

Prep Time: 5 minutes

Cook Time: 10 minutes

Directions:

✓ In a saucepan, combine beef broth and drippings.
✓ Bring to a simmer and cook until thickened.
✓ Season with salt and pepper.

Nutritional Information: Calories: 30, Protein: 0g, Fat: 3g (per tablespoon)

LEMON BUTTER SAUCE

Ingredients: 1/2 cup butter, 1 tbsp lemon juice, salt.

Prep Time: 5 minutes

Cook Time: 5 minutes

Directions:

- ✓ Melt the butter in a saucepan.
- ✓ Stir in lemon juice and salt.
- ✓ Serve over seafood or chicken.

Nutritional Information: Calories: 102, Protein: 0g, Fat: 11g (per tablespoon)

SPICY MUSTARD SAUCE

Ingredients: 1/4 cup mustard, 1/4 cup mayonnaise, 1 tsp hot sauce, salt.

Prep Time: 5 minutes

Cook Time: 0 minutes

Directions:

- ✓ Mix mustard, mayonnaise, hot sauce, and salt.
- ✓ Adjust the hot sauce to your desired level of spiciness.

Nutritional Information: Calories: 100, Protein: 0g, Fat: 11g (per tablespoon)

GARLIC AIOLI

Ingredients: 1 egg yolk, 3/4 cup olive oil, 1 clove garlic, minced, 1 tsp lemon juice, salt.

Prep Time: 10 minutes

Cook Time: 0 minutes

Directions:

- ✓ Whisk the egg yolk with lemon juice, garlic, and salt.
- ✓ Slowly drizzle in the olive oil, whisking continuously until thickened.

Nutritional Information: Calories: 100, Protein: 0g, Fat: 11g (per tablespoon)

ANCHOVY BUTTER

Ingredients: 1/2 cup butter, 4 anchovy fillets, minced.

Prep Time: 5 minutes

Cook Time: 0 minutes

Directions:

- ✓ Mix softened butter with minced anchovies.
- ✓ Use as a spread or to melt over grilled meats.

Nutritional Information: Calories: 102, Protein: 1g, Fat: 11g (per tablespoon)

BACON JAM

Ingredients: 1 lb. bacon, 1/4 cup brewed coffee, 1 tbsp apple cider vinegar, salt.

Prep Time: 10 minutes

Cook Time: 1 hour

Directions:

- ✓ Cook bacon until crispy.
- ✓ Chop and return to the pan with coffee and vinegar.
- ✓ Simmer until thickened.
- ✓ Season with salt.

Nutritional Information: Calories: 60, Protein: 4g, Fat: 4g (per tablespoon)

CHIMICHURRI (CARNIVORE VERSION)

Ingredients: 1/2 cup beef tallow, 2 tbsp dried parsley, 2 tbsp dried oregano, 1 tsp garlic powder, 1 tbsp red wine vinegar, salt, and pepper.

Prep Time: 5 minutes

Cook Time: 0 minutes

Directions:

- ✓ Mix melted beef tallow with dried parsley, oregano, garlic powder, vinegar, salt, and pepper.
- ✓ Serve with grilled meats.

Nutritional Information: Calories: 100, Protein: 0g, Fat: 11g (per tablespoon)

CREAMY BLUE CHEESE DRESSING

Ingredients: 1/2 cup sour cream, 1/4 cup crumbled blue cheese, 1 tbsp mayonnaise, salt, and pepper.

Prep Time: 5 minutes

Cook Time: 0 minutes

Directions:

- ✓ Mix sour cream, blue cheese, mayonnaise, salt, and pepper.
- ✓ Adjust the amount of blue cheese to taste.

Nutritional Information: Calories: 60, Protein: 1g, Fat: 6g (per tablespoon)

HOLLANDAISE SAUCE

Ingredients: 3 egg yolks, 1/2 cup melted butter, 1 tbsp lemon juice, salt.

Prep Time: 5 minutes

Cook Time: 5 minutes

Directions:

- ✓ Whisk egg yolks and lemon juice over low heat until thickened.
- ✓ Slowly whisk in melted butter.
- ✓ Season with salt.

Nutritional Information: Calories: 102, Protein: 1g, Fat: 11g (per tablespoon)

CAVIAR CREAM

Ingredients: 1/4 cup sour cream, 2 tbsp caviar, salt.

Prep Time: 5 minutes

Cook Time: 0 minutes

Directions:

- ✓ Mix sour cream and caviar.
- ✓ Season with salt.
- ✓ Serve as a topping for blinis or steak.

Nutritional Information: Calories: 25, Protein: 1g, Fat: 2g (per tablespoon)

BÉARNAISE SAUCE

Ingredients: 3 egg yolks, 1/2 cup melted butter, 1 tbsp tarragon vinegar, 1 tbsp minced tarragon, salt.

Prep Time: 5 minutes

Cook Time: 5 minutes

Directions:

- ✓ Whisk egg yolks and vinegar over low heat until thickened.
- ✓ Slowly whisk in melted butter.
- ✓ Stir in minced tarragon and season with salt.

Nutritional Information: Calories: 102, Protein: 1g, Fat: 11g (per tablespoon)

TRUFFLE BUTTER

Ingredients: 1/2 cup butter, 1 tbsp truffle oil, salt.

Prep Time: 5 minutes

Cook Time: 0 minutes

Directions:

- ✓ Mix softened butter with truffle oil and salt.

✓ Use as a spread or to melt over grilled meats.

Nutritional Information: Calories: 102, Protein: 0g, Fat: 11g (per tablespoon)

Every single one of these sauces and condiments are meant to offer extra nutrition to your carnivore diet meals while also improving their flavor. These recipes provide a range of options to meet the nutritional needs and taste preferences, perhaps you're searching for a sour and spicy condiment or a rich and creamy sauce.

CHAPTER 14:

CARNIVORE DIET MEAL PLANNING

To retain social life and guarantee adequate nutrition, following the Carnivore Diet involves cautious planning and preparation. The following guide offers detailed instructions for planning meals on a daily and weekly basis, controlling eating out, controlling portion sizes, grocery shopping, preparing meals, and conquering cravings and cheat days.

Daily and Weekly Meal Plans

Organizing your meals is essential to following the Carnivore Diet. The following advice can be used to make weekly and daily meal plans:

Start with a Template: Outline your meals for the day, including breakfast, lunch, dinner, and any snacks. Repeat this process for the entire week.

Incorporate Variety: Rotate different types of meat and animal products throughout the week to ensure a diverse nutrient intake. Include beef, pork, poultry, fish, organ meats, and eggs.

Balance Your Macros: Achieve a good balance between fat and protein in each meal. For instance, serve fish or chicken breast alongside a slimmer cut of steak.

Plan for Leftovers: Make more food to freeze for later use or to have leftovers for the next day. Meal preparation time and effort are reduced as a result.

Breakfast: Chicken Liver Pâté - Spread on thin slices of crispy bacon.

Lunch: Grilled T-Bone Steak - Seasoned lightly and grilled to desired doneness.

Dinner: Beef Heart Skewers - Cubed, seasoned, and grilled, served with a side of homemade aioli.

Snack: Pork Rinds - Light and crispy, seasoned with salt.

SUNDAY

Breakfast: Fried Chicken Gizzards - Tender gizzards fried until crispy and golden.

Lunch: Seared Tuna Steaks - Just a hint of sesame oil and seared to preserve the freshness of the fish.

Dinner: Roasted Bone Marrow - Roasted with a sprinkle of sea salt, scooped straight from the bone.

Snack: Deviled Eggs - Made with a creamy filling and a dash of paprika.

Tips for Eating Out and Social Situations

Going to social gatherings or eating out can be difficult when following the Carnivore Diet. Here are different approaches for dealing similar conditions:

Research Restaurants: Search internet menus for items that appeal to carnivores, such barbecue places or steakhouses.

Communicate Your Needs: Don't hesitate to ask for modifications to your order, such as substituting side dishes with extra meat or requesting sauces and dressings on the side.

Bring Your Own Food: If attending a social event, consider bringing your own carnivore-approved dish to share.

Stay Focused: Keep in mind your nutritional objectives and the basis for your decision to follow the carnivore diet. This can assist you in overcoming the want to deviate from your goal.

Portion Size and Frequency

To stay full and achieve your nutritional needs, it's necessary to comprehend portion sizes and meal timing:

Listen to Your Body: When you are hungry, eat, and when you are satisfied, stop. Since the Carnivore Diet naturally satisfies, you could discover that you eat less frequently in general.

Adjust Portions Based on Activity Level: If you're more active, you may need larger portions or more frequent meals to fuel your energy needs.

Use Visual Cues: A serving of beef is typically approximately the size of your hand or a deck of cards. Adapt to your signals of hunger and fullness.

Tips for Grocery Shopping and Meal Prep

Following the Carnivore Diet can be easier to manage if groceries are purchased and meals are prepared efficiently:

Make a List: Make a grocery list based on your meal plan to make sure you have everything you need and to help you resist impulsive purchases.

Shop the Perimeter: Pay attention to the areas around the fresh meats and animal goods that are usually seen in the grocery store.

Batch Cook: To save time over the week, prepare large amounts of meat at once. For example, roast an entire chicken or grill several steaks.

Store Properly: Cooked meats should be kept in the freezer or refrigerator in airtight containers to preserve freshness and avoid spoiling.

How to Handle Cravings and Cheat Days

When starting a new diet, cravings and the urge for cheat days are typical. These are some pointers for handling these difficulties:

Identify Triggers: Acknowledge the factors that are responsible for your wants, which may include social cues, boredom, or stress. Developing coping strategies for particular stimuli can help reduce cravings.

Stay Hydrated: Sometimes thirst is mistaken for hunger. Drinking water can help curb cravings.

Eat Satiating Meals: To stave off hunger and cravings, make sure your meals are filling and high in nutrients.

Plan for Cheat Days: If you do choose to indulge in a cheat day, schedule it ahead of time and establish rules for yourself. This can facilitate the transition back to your carnivorous habit and help avoid overindulgence.

Be Kind to Yourself: Don't be too hard on yourself if you give in to a craving or take a day off. Recognize it, take what you can from it, and proceed.

The Carnivore Diet calls for organized daily and weekly food planning, social scenario management, portion control awareness, effective grocery shopping and meal preparation, and control over cravings and cheat days. You may follow the Carnivore Diet and reap its benefits if you prepare ahead and have a positive outlook.

CHAPTER 15:

CARNIVORE COOKING TECHNIQUES: MASTERING THE ART OF MEAT PREPARATION

To begin a carnivorous diet, one must not only know what kinds of meat to eat, but also how to prepare it such that each meal is nutrient-dense and tastes excellent. This guide focuses toward the art of meat preparation, providing both new and seasoned meat lovers with an extensive introduction. Sous vide, grilling, smoking, and repurposing leftovers are among the topics discussed.

1. Grilling: The Quintessential Carnivore Cooking Method

Meats are pleasantly charred and given a smokey flavor by grilling, which is a basic and primeval technique. From steaks and burgers to ribs and kebabs, it works well with a wide range of meats.

Choosing the Right Cut: Choose for grilling pieces like T-bone steaks, sirloin, or rib eye that have a nice ratio of muscle to fat. Since they keep more of their juice, thicker cuts are preferred.

Preparation: The meat should be room temperature and thoroughly dried before being grilled. Salt and pepper, if preferred, should be added liberally. Flare-ups can be avoided by avoiding marinades that include too much liquid or sugar.

Grilling Technique: Set the grill to high heat. After putting the meat on the grill, leave it alone for a few minutes to sear. Flip it once with tongs so that each side has a beautiful crust. To finish cooking thicker pieces indirectly, move them to a cooler area of the grill.

Doneness: To make sure the meat is the right doneness, use a meat thermometer. The usual ranges for uncommon are 120–130°F, medium–rare 130–135°F, and medium 135–145°F. To preserve the fluids, let the meat rest for a few minutes before slicing.

2. Smoking: Infusing Depth and Flavor

Meats are given a rich, earthy flavor by smoking, a low-and-slow cooking technique. It works well with tougher pieces like ribs, pork shoulder, and brisket that benefit from lengthy cooking durations.

Choosing Wood: Different flavors are imparted by different timbers. Apple and cherry are softer and sweeter than hickory and mesquite, which are powerful and forceful. Try different things to see what you like.

Preparation: Rub some salt and spices on the meat in a basic dry rub. If you want to add more taste and moisture to larger chunks, you might want to consider injecting with a brine solution.

Smoking Technique: Preheat the smoker to 225-250°F. Place the meat in the smoker, ensuring it's not directly over the heat source. Maintain a consistent temperature and replenish wood chips as needed.

Patience is Key: Depending on the size and cut, smoking may take many hours. Check the doneness of the meat with a meat thermometer. Brisket, for instance, is usually cooked between 195 and 205°F.

3. Sous Vide: Precision and Perfection

The French cooking method known as "sous vide" entails vacuum-sealing meat in a bag and bringing it to a precise temperature in a water bath. It's the best way to get the appropriate amount of fragility and doneness.

Equipment: You'll need a sous vide precision cooker and vacuum-seal bags. The cooker circulates and heats the water, maintaining a consistent temperature.

Preparation: Season the meat and place it in a vacuum-seal bag. Remove as much air as possible and seal the bag.

Cooking Technique: Ascertain the ideal temperature for your meat cut in the water bath. For a medium-rare steak, for instance, 130°F. Close the bag and submerge it in the water. Cook for the specified amount of time (up to 24 hours for harder cuts, or 1 hour for steaks).

Finishing Touch: After sous vide cooking, sear the meat quickly in a hot pan or on a grill to develop a flavorful crust.

4. Making the Most of Leftovers

Leftovers from the carnivore diet can be transformed into scrumptious new dishes, saving time and minimizing waste.

Reinventing Meals: Turn leftover steak into a hearty salad topping, or shred leftover roast beef for a savory omelet filling. Leftover chicken can be diced and added to a broth for a simple soup.

Storage: Store leftovers properly in airtight containers in the refrigerator. Most cooked meats can be safely stored for 3-4 days.

Safety: Reheat leftovers to an internal temperature of 165°F to ensure safety. Use a meat thermometer to check.

You may make your meals more fulfilling and nutritious by learning these carnivorous cooking techniques, which will also expand your culinary skills. The secret is to appreciate the food and have fun while cooking, the fact that you're smoking a soft brisket, sous videing an ideal filet, or inventively using leftovers. You'll gain a deeper understanding of the art of meat preparation and the carnivore lifestyle via experimentation and practice.

CHAPTER 16:

CARNIVORE DIET STYLES AND RECOMMENDATIONS

With its emphasis on foods derived from animals, the Carnivore Diet offers a variety of strategies to accommodate various health objectives, tastes, and lifestyles. This book explores the many forms of carnivore eating, offers advice on how to modify the diet to suit your preferences, and suggests ways to maximize wellbeing.

1. Different Approaches to Carnivore Eating

There is no one-size-fits-all Carnivore Diet; instead, it can be customized to meet the needs and tastes of each person. These are a few typical variations:

Strict Carnivore: This approach involves consuming only meat, primarily from ruminant animals like beef, lamb, and bison. It excludes all plant foods, dairy, and processed meats.

Nose-to-Tail Carnivore: Emphasizing nutrient density, this style includes not only muscle meats but also organ meats, bone marrow, and animal fats. It aims to utilize all parts of the animal for a broader spectrum of nutrients.

Keto Carnivore: Similar to a ketogenic diet, this variation improves the fat-to-protein ratio in order to encourage ketosis. In order to boost fat consumption, it permits a moderate intake of milk and other dairy goods like butter and heavy cream.

Dairy-Inclusive Carnivore: For those who tolerate dairy well, this style includes cheese, butter, and heavy cream, providing additional fat sources and variety in the diet.

Seafood-Heavy Carnivore: This approach emphasizes fish and other seafood, which are rich in omega-3 fatty acids, alongside traditional meat sources.

2. Tailoring the Diet to Your Needs

To make the Carnivore Diet work for you, consider the following factors:

Health Goals: You may concentrate on leaner meat cuts and watch your calorie intake if you're trying to lose weight. Eat more foods high in protein if you want to gain muscle, and plan your meals around your workouts.

Food Tolerances: Observe how your body responds to various foods. While some people may discover that specific varieties of meat suit them better, others may need to limit or avoid dairy altogether.

Nutritional Needs: Ensure you're getting a balanced intake of nutrients. Incorporating organ meats can help cover your vitamin and mineral requirements.

Lifestyle and Preferences: Consider your budget, cooking skills, and taste preferences. The diet should be sustainable and enjoyable for you.

3. Recommendations for Optimal Health

To maximize the benefits of the Carnivore Diet, keep these recommendations in mind:

Prioritize Quality: Pick animal products that have been grown on pasture, fed grass, or captured in the wild whenever feasible. Higher nutrient content and absence of additional hormones and antibiotics are characteristic of these.

Stay Hydrated: Water is your best beverage throughout the day. For additional minerals and electrolytes, think about adding bone broth.

Manage Electrolytes: Add salt to taste and, if necessary, think about taking magnesium and potassium supplements, especially in the early stages of adaptation.

Listen to Your Body: Adjust your food intake based on hunger and satiety signals. The Carnivore Diet can naturally regulate appetite, so trust your body's cues.

Experiment with Fasting: Many carnivores find that intermittent fasting or time-restricted eating comes naturally and can enhance the diet's benefits.

Monitor Your Health: Pay attention to your digestion, energy, and general health. Monitoring changes in your health markers might be facilitated by routine blood testing.

Stay Active: Incorporate regular physical activity to complement the diet and support muscle health, cardiovascular fitness, and mental well-being.

Be Patient: It may take some time to make the switch to a carnivorous diet, particularly if you're coming from a typical American or high-carb diet. Allow your body to adjust over time.

Seek Support: Connect with others on the carnivore diet through social media, forums, or local groups. Sharing experiences and tips can be invaluable.

To accommodate a range of requirements and tastes, the Carnivore Diet offers multiple variations. By being aware of the many methods, customizing the diet to meet your needs, and adhering to the main guidelines, you may reap the rewards of this meat-centric diet while also improving your health. Even if you are a new or seasoned carnivore, a successful and lasting journey can be achieved by implementing this diet with awareness and flexibility.

CHAPTER 17:

CARNIVORE DIET FOR ATHLETES AND BODYBUILDERS: ENHANCING PERFORMANCE AND RECOVERY

Athletes and bodybuilders have come to love the Carnivore Diet because of its supposed advantages for recuperation and performance. This thorough book covers important issues for athletes, how to include a carnivorous diet into a training program, and how to optimize the diet for athletic performance.

1. Performance and Recovery on a Carnivore Diet

Protein for Muscle Growth and Repair: For bodybuilders and athletes hoping to gain and preserve muscle mass, the high protein intake of the carnivore diet facilitates muscle synthesis. All of the essential amino acids required for muscle growth and repair are found in animal proteins.

Fat as a Fuel Source: On a carnivore diet, the body adapts to using fat as its primary energy source. This metabolic shift can enhance endurance by tapping into the body's fat reserves for sustained energy, reducing reliance on carbohydrates.

Reduced Inflammation: The body's inflammation may decrease as a result of cutting out plant-based diets, which may have anti-nutrients and inflammatory chemicals. Recoveries more quickly and overall sports performance can be improved by reduced inflammation.

Improved Joint Health: The emphasis on collagen-rich foods like bone broth and connective tissues can support joint health, essential for athletes engaging in high-impact activities.

Enhanced Nutrient Absorption: Highly accessible forms of vital minerals, like as iron, zinc, and B vitamins, are provided by a carnivorous diet. These nutrients are critical for the creation of energy and general athletic performance.

2. Specific Considerations for Athletes

Energy Requirements: Because they work so hard, bodybuilders and athletes may require more energy. To support exercise and recuperation, you must eat enough calories, mostly from fat and protein.

Protein Intake: Although the carnivore diet is centered around protein, athletes should make sure they're getting enough of it to support muscle growth and repair. Eating more food that is high in protein, such as seafood and organ meats, or eating larger portions may be necessary to achieve this.

Hydration and Electrolytes: Drinking enough of water is essential, particularly when the body is adjusting to a carnivorous diet and may lose more electrolytes and water. Athletes should be aware of their level of hydration and, if needed, think about taking an electrolyte supplement.

Pre- and Post-Workout Nutrition: Timing nutrient intake around workouts can optimize performance and recovery. Consuming easily digestible....le protein and fat before training can provide sustained energy, while a protein-rich meal post-workout can aid in muscle recovery.

Adaptation Period: There may be a period of adaptation when switching to a carnivorous diet during which time athletic performance may temporarily decline. Athletes should regularly monitor their performance and give their bodies time to acclimate to the new fuel source.

Flexibility for Carb-Loading: A planned carb loading regimen prior to tournaments or rigorous training sessions may be beneficial for certain athletes. Small amounts of carbs like honey or dairy might give you a brief energy boost without taking too much away from the carnivorous model.

Monitoring Health Markers: Regular blood work and health check-ups can help athletes monitor their response to the diet and make adjustments as needed to ensure optimal performance and health.

3. Integrating the Carnivore Diet into an Athletic Lifestyle

Gradual Transition: To avoid possible disturbances to their training, athletes might think about easing into a carnivorous diet. This can be done by starting with a low-carb or ketogenic diet and gradually removing plant foods.

Variety for Nutrient Density: Incorporating a variety of animal-based foods, including muscle meats, organ meats, and seafood, can ensure a wide range of nutrients to support athletic performance.

Experimentation with Macros: Experimenting with different macronutrient ratios can help athletes find the optimal balance for their energy needs and performance goals.

Listening to the Body: Athletes should pay close attention to their body's signals, adjusting their diet and training based on how they feel and perform.

In order to improve recuperation and performance, this innovative approach to bodybuilding and sports nutrition strongly emphasizes foods high in nutrients derived from animals. Athletes can tailor this diet to meet their training and competition objectives by taking into account their unique calorie requirements, making sure they consume enough protein, and keeping an eye on their hydration and electrolyte levels. Athletes can successfully adopt a carnivore diet by implementing a gradual transition, closely monitoring health markers, and seeking professional counsel, just like they can with any dietary adjustment.

CHAPTER 18:
CARNIVORE DIET AND WEIGHT MANAGEMENT

With its sole emphasis on meals derived from animals, the Carnivore Diet has become increasingly well-liked as a weight-loss strategy. The carnivore diet is a popular method for losing weight and promoting health, and in this article, we'll examine its foundational ideas and offer tips and tactics suitable for novices as well as veteran users.

1. Using the Carnivore Diet for Fat Loss

Simplicity and Satiety: The carnivorous diet makes eating easier and lowers the risk of overindulging. Rich in fat and protein, two very satiating macronutrients, animal-based diets can help suppress appetite and cut back on overall calorie consumption.

Metabolic Advantage: The carnivore diet causes the body to enter a state of ketosis, when it burns fat rather than glucose for energy, by removing carbs from the diet. This metabolic state, especially in conjunction with a calorie deficit, can improve fat reduction.

Protein's Role in Fat Loss: Protein digests more energy-densely than fats or carbs because it has a significant thermic impact. A higher metabolic rate and weight reduction may result from this increased energy expenditure.

Hormonal Regulation: Hormones linked to controlling weight can benefit from a carnivorous diet. To help manage appetite and lose fat, it could, for instance, increase insulin sensitivity and lower levels of the hunger hormone ghrelin.

2. Maintaining a Healthy Weight on Carnivore

Listening to Your Body: Observe your body's signals of hunger and fullness. Since the carnivore diet naturally controls hunger, eating until full rather than overindulging can support weight maintenance.

Monitoring Weight and Body Composition: You can maintain your target weight by modifying your diet as necessary by keeping a regular record of your weight and body composition. Keep in mind that variations are typical and concentrate on long-term patterns.

Incorporating Physical Activity: Strength training in particular can help sustain muscle growth and a healthy metabolism in addition to a carnivorous diet. Maintaining a healthy weight over time requires doing this.

Adapting to Energy Needs: You may need to modify your consumption of fat and protein as you enter your weight maintenance phase in order to meet your energy requirements. For weight maintenance, some people can find it helpful to modestly increase their diet of fat.

3. Considerations for Long Term Success

Nutrient Density: To make sure you're getting all the micronutrients you need while keeping a healthy weight, give nutrient-dense animal foods like organ meats and fatty fish first priority.

Addressing Plateaus: Plateaus in weight loss are typical. If you find yourself stuck, think about boosting your exercise, trying with intermittent fasting, or modifying your calorie consumption.

Psychological Aspects: It's critical to keep up a positive relationship with food. Steer clear of compulsive calorie counting and concentrate on providing your body with superior animal-based nutrition.

Individual Variability: Everybody reacts to dietary changes differently in their body. To determine what macronutrient ratios and meal selections are ideal for you, have patience and be open to trying new things.

Medical Supervision: If you have any underlying health conditions or concerns, it's important to work with a healthcare professional to ensure the carnivore diet is appropriate for your individual health needs.

With its straightforward and satisfying eating strategy, the diet based on meat and poultry can be a useful tool for managing weight. You can adopt the carnivore diet to attain and maintain a healthy weight by emphasizing nutrient-dense animal-based meals, paying attention to your body's signals, and engaging in regular physical activity. During your weight-loss journey, don't forget to track your progress, be flexible, and put your general health and well-being first.

CHAPTER 19:

CARNIVORE DIET: FREQUENTLY ASKED QUESTIONS

Because the Carnivore Diet emphasizes items derived from animals, it frequently prompts a lot of queries and worries. We try to answer the most often asked questions in this section of the book, offering concise and thorough explanations for anyone who wants to know more about the carnivore diet.

1. What can I eat on the Carnivore Diet?

Answer: On the Carnivore Diet, you can eat meat, fish, eggs, and animal-derived products like butter and lard. This includes beef, pork, chicken, lamb, organ meats, seafood, and shellfish. Dairy is allowed for some individuals, depending on tolerance.

2. Is the Carnivore Diet safe?

Answer: The Carnivore Diet can be safe for many people, especially in the short term. However, long-term effects are less understood. It's important to monitor nutrient intake and consult with a healthcare professional, especially if you have existing health conditions.

3. How does the Carnivore Diet affect cholesterol levels?

Answer: The Carnivore Diet may increase LDL ("bad") cholesterol in some individuals, but it can also raise HDL ("good") cholesterol. The impact on heart health is still debated, and individual responses vary. Regular monitoring of lipid profiles is recommended.

4. Can I lose weight on the Carnivore Diet?

Answer: Yes, many people experience weight loss on the Carnivore Diet due to its high protein content, which promotes satiety, and the elimination of processed foods and carbohydrates.

5. How do I get enough vitamins and minerals on the Carnivore Diet?

Answer: Animal foods, especially organ meats, are rich in vitamins and minerals. To ensure adequate nutrient intake, include a variety of meats, organ meats, and seafood in your diet.

6. Will I experience constipation on the Carnivore Diet?

Answer: Some individuals may experience constipation when transitioning to the Carnivore Diet, often due to reduced fiber intake. Staying hydrated and incorporating organ meats can help alleviate this issue.

7. Is the Carnivore Diet suitable for athletes?

Answer: Yes, the Carnivore Diet can be suitable for athletes, providing ample protein for muscle repair and growth. However, athletes may need to adjust their fat and protein intake based on their energy expenditure and performance goals.

8. Can I drink coffee or tea on the Carnivore Diet?

Answer: While purists may exclude them, many people on the Carnivore Diet allow beverages like coffee and tea. It ultimately depends on individual tolerance and preference.

9. How do I avoid nutrient deficiencies on the Carnivore Diet?

Answer: To avoid nutrient deficiencies, focus on consuming a variety of animal-based foods, including muscle meats, organ meats, and fatty fish, which provide a wide range of essential nutrients.

9. Can the Carnivore Diet improve gut health?
10.

Answer: Some proponents claim that the Carnivore Diet can improve gut health by eliminating plant-based foods that may cause irritation or inflammation in certain individuals. However, more research is needed in this area.

11. How does the Carnivore Diet impact mental health?

Answer: Anecdotal reports suggest that the Carnivore Diet may improve mental clarity and mood in some individuals, possibly due to its potential anti-inflammatory effects. However, scientific evidence is limited.

12. Is the Carnivore Diet sustainable long-term?

Answer: The sustainability of the Carnivore Diet long-term is debated. While some individuals thrive on this diet indefinitely, others may need to reintroduce certain plant foods or supplements to maintain optimal health.

13. How do I transition to the Carnivore Diet?

Answer: To transition to the Carnivore Diet, gradually reduce your intake of plant-based foods while increasing your consumption of animal-based foods. Pay attention to your body's responses and adjust accordingly.

14. Can I follow the Carnivore Diet if I have a chronic health condition?

Answer: If you have a chronic health condition, it's crucial to consult with a healthcare professional before starting the Carnivore Diet. The diet may need to be modified to suit your specific health needs.

15. How do I ensure I'm eating enough on the Carnivore Diet?

Answer: Listen to your body's hunger and satiety cues. The Carnivore Diet naturally regulates appetite, so eat until you are satisfied. If you're concerned about under-eating, track your food intake and adjust as needed.

The Carnivore Diet poses a number of queries and worries, ranging from dietary consumption and safety to its effects on managing weight and long-term medical disorders. People can make well-informed decisions and customize their diets to meet their own requirements and objectives by answering these often-asked questions. As with any dietary plan, it's critical to pay attention to your health, listen to your body, and seek professional advice when needed.

CONCLUSION AND MOVING FORWARD:

The transition to a carnivorous lifestyle involves a significant change in eating habits and a return to the most basic elements of nutrition. It is a transforming and personal experience. As we come to the end of this in-depth examination of the carnivore diet, it's important to think back on the fundamental ideas that guide this eating style and how one might stay healthy while following it.

Embracing the Carnivore Lifestyle

Simplicity and Focus: The carnivore diet is fundamentally about focus and simplicity. It returns to the fundamentals of animal-based nutrition by dissecting the complexity of contemporary food options. It might be freeing to focus less on tracking calories or macros and more on the quality of your diet thanks to its simplicity.

Listening to Your Body: The carnivorous diet promotes a keen awareness of your body's cues. Take note of how different foods make you feel and use that information to modify your diet. A more peaceful relationship with food and eating can result from using this intuitive technique.

Prioritizing Quality: Stress how crucial it is to get nutrient-dense, premium animal meals. Seafood that is obtained in the wild, meats that have been reared on pasture, and organic eggs are all excellent options that can promote sustainable farming methods and offer a wider variety of nutrients.

Respecting Individuality: Understand that there is no one-size-fits-all method for implementing a carnivorous diet. Individual requirements and reactions differ, therefore it's critical to customize the diet to your particular situation, whether that is introducing particular dairy products, experimenting with organ meats, or modifying the proportions of fat to protein.

Continuing Your Carnivore Journey

Ongoing Learning and Adaptation: The carnivore diet is a journey of continuous learning and adaptation. Stay informed about the latest research and developments in the field, and be open to refining your approach as you gain new insights and experiences.

Community and Support: Interacting with the carnivore community can be a great way to get inspiration and support. Making connections with people who are on a similar path, whether through social media, online forums, or local groups, can provide support, knowledge sharing, and a feeling of community.

Holistic Health Focus: Although diet plays a major role, it's imperative to take a holistic approach to health. To enhance the benefits of a carnivore diet, add in regular physical activity, give sleep and stress management first priority, and take care of your mental and emotional health.

Long-Term Sustainability: Think about how sustainable the carnivorous lifestyle is in the long run. This covers concerns about animal sourcing and eating from an ethical and environmental standpoint in addition to personal health and well-being.

Navigating Challenges: Be ready to triumph over obstacles and disappointments. Having plans in place for tackling social situations, taking care of dietary issues, and controlling cravings can all help you stay dedicated to your carnivorous path.

Celebrating Successes: Celebrate and acknowledge your small victories along the way. Acknowledging your accomplishments can inspire you to keep going, whether it's through better health indicators, increased physical performance, or a renewed sense of energy.

In order to wrap up, adopting a carnivorous lifestyle involves more than just changing your food. It's about listening to your body, reestablishing ancestors' dietary habits, and making wise choices that promote your overall health and wellbeing. As you proceed, keep in mind that the carnivore diet is a way of life that respects the simplicity, wisdom, and sustenance of nature rather than merely a method of eating.

THANK YOU FOR YOUR TRUST AND TIME!

WE HOPE YOU ENJOYED YOUR EXPERIENCE WITH OUR CARNIVORE CODE COOKBOOK. YOUR FEEDBACK IS NOT JUST IMPORTANT TO US—IT'S VITAL. IT HELPS US UNDERSTAND YOUR NEEDS BETTER AND MAKES A REAL DIFFERENCE IN HOW WE IMPROVE AND EVOLVE.

COULD YOU TAKE A MOMENT TO SHARE YOUR THOUGHTS? AN HONEST REVIEW FROM YOU WOULD MEAN THE WORLD TO US AND HELPS OTHERS MAKE INFORMED DECISIONS. PLUS, WE LOVE HEARING HOW WE CAN MAKE YOUR EXPERIENCE EVEN MORE REMARKABLE NEXT TIME!

WELCOME TO THE CARNIVOROUS LIFESTYLE

WEEKLY MEAL PLANNER

MONDAY

BREAKFAST_______________________

LUNCH_______________________

DINNER_______________________

SNACKS_______________________

TUESDAY

BREAKFAST_______________________

LUNCH_______________________

DINNER_______________________

SNACKS_______________________

WEDNESDAY

BREAKFAST_______________________

LUNCH_______________________

DINNER_______________________

SNACKS_______________________

THURSDAY

BREAKFAST_______________________

LUNCH_______________________

DINNER_______________________

SNACKS_______________________

FRIDAY

BREAKFAST_______________________

LUNCH_______________________

DINNER_______________________

SNACKS_______________________

SATURDAY

BREAKFAST_______________________

LUNCH_______________________

DINNER_______________________

SNACKS_______________________

SUNDAY

BREAKFAST_______________________

LUNCH_______________________

DINNER_______________________

SNACKS_______________________

NOTES

____

____

____

____

WEEKLY MEAL PLANNER

MONDAY

BREAKFAST_______________________

LUNCH_______________________

DINNER_______________________

SNACKS_______________________

TUESDAY

BREAKFAST_______________________

LUNCH_______________________

DINNER_______________________

SNACKS_______________________

WEDNESDAY

BREAKFAST_______________________

LUNCH_______________________

DINNER_______________________

SNACKS_______________________

THURSDAY

BREAKFAST_______________________

LUNCH_______________________

DINNER_______________________

SNACKS_______________________

FRIDAY

BREAKFAST_______________________

LUNCH_______________________

DINNER_______________________

SNACKS_______________________

SATURDAY

BREAKFAST_______________________

LUNCH_______________________

DINNER_______________________

SNACKS_______________________

SUNDAY

BREAKFAST_______________________

LUNCH_______________________

DINNER_______________________

SNACKS_______________________

NOTES

____

____

____

____

____

WEEKLY MEAL PLANNER

MONDAY

BREAKFAST

LUNCH

DINNER

SNACKS

TUESDAY

BREAKFAST

LUNCH

DINNER

SNACKS

WEDNESDAY

BREAKFAST

LUNCH

DINNER

SNACKS

THURSDAY

BREAKFAST

LUNCH

DINNER

SNACKS

FRIDAY

BREAKFAST

LUNCH

DINNER

SNACKS

SATURDAY

BREAKFAST

LUNCH

DINNER

SNACKS

SUNDAY

BREAKFAST

LUNCH

DINNER

SNACKS

NOTES

WEEKLY MEAL PLANNER

MONDAY

BREAKFAST_______________________

LUNCH_______________________

DINNER_______________________

SNACKS_______________________

TUESDAY

BREAKFAST_______________________

LUNCH_______________________

DINNER_______________________

SNACKS_______________________

WEDNESDAY

BREAKFAST_______________________

LUNCH_______________________

DINNER_______________________

SNACKS_______________________

THURSDAY

BREAKFAST_______________________

LUNCH_______________________

DINNER_______________________

SNACKS_______________________

FRIDAY

BREAKFAST_______________________

LUNCH_______________________

DINNER_______________________

SNACKS_______________________

SATURDAY

BREAKFAST_______________________

LUNCH_______________________

DINNER_______________________

SNACKS_______________________

SUNDAY

BREAKFAST_______________________

LUNCH_______________________

DINNER_______________________

SNACKS_______________________

NOTES

____

____

____

____

____

NOTES